‘This book should be required reading for all therapists. Its contributors put words to the unspeakable and bear witness to the unbearable. No human being can fully represent the horrors and continuing psychological depredations of war, and yet these essays manage to capture the precariousness and preciousness of our existence, the power of our feelings about place, and the critical role of our moral center of gravity in the face of evil. With clarity, passion, and brilliance, these authors help us see that although war-adapted psychotherapies can help only in modest ways, they matter profoundly.’

Nancy McWilliams, *PhD, ABPP, visiting professor Emerita, Rutgers Graduate School of Applied & Professional Psychology*

‘The urgency of this book, both for those who live under conditions of war and for psychoanalysis itself, cannot be overstated. In this volume’s efforts to un-silence, in real time, the consequences of the ongoing Russian effort to annihilate individuals, culture and country and is a quintessential antidote to war’s dehumanizing force and demanding of us that we embrace the possibilities inherent in our profession. The valuable opportunity this volume provides melds theory, practice and personal experience to expand our clinical, conceptual and moral capacities to counter the violent occupation that so much of our world is seemingly authorized by fascism’s rise to perpetuate. There is a testimony here to the isomorphic interchange between psychic and large-group catastrophe, but there is also, in this series of essays, much hope and inspiration in the authors’ persistence in speaking psychoanalytically-informed truth, to which it behooves us to listen, despite all.’

Nancy Burke, *PhD, ABPP, clinical professor, Northwestern University, Chicago Center for Psychoanalysis*

Psychoanalytic Practices and Russia's War Against Ukraine

This book looks at the impact of multigenerational trauma, severe psychopathology, and ethical struggles through the lens of Ukrainian psychoanalysts working amidst the Russian invasion.

The contribution examines psychoanalytic responses to Russia's aggression against Ukraine, including via lived experiences of Ukrainian psychoanalysts who practice under conditions of continued threat. The book offers analytic observations and exploration of psychoanalytically informed care with Ukrainians who are experiencing profound distress and war trauma. Contributors describe their work with diverse Ukrainian groups, including children and adolescents, war refugees, individuals experiencing severe physical and psychological crises, Ukrainian Jewish community, and Ukrainian diaspora.

This will be a valuable resource for readers interested in understanding and responding to impact of wars, specifically genocidal wars. They are invited to witness the profound challenges, creativity, courage, human and professional dilemmas, and pain that are witnessed and responded to by psychoanalytically informed practitioners.

Mariana Velykodna is a EuroPsy-registered psychologist, psychoanalytic psychotherapist certified by the European Confederation of Psychoanalytic Psychotherapies, an associate professor and Head of Psychoanalytic Psychotherapy Department at Ukraine Sigmund Freud University in Ukraine.

Oksana Yakushko is a licensed psychologist, psychoanalyst, and Ukrainian immigrant. She is a faculty at the George Washington University and a psychoanalytic practitioner in California and Washington, DC.

Adrienne Harris is a faculty and supervisor in the New York University Postdoctoral Program in Psychotherapy and Psychoanalysis, Faculty and Training analyst at the Psychoanalytic Institute of Northern California, and serves on Editorial Boards of several psychoanalytic journals.

Relational Perspectives Book Series

The Relational Perspectives Book Series (RPBS) publishes books that grow out of or contribute to the relational tradition in contemporary psychoanalysis. The term *relational psychoanalysis* was first used by Greenberg and Mitchell[1] to bridge the traditions of interpersonal relations, as developed within interpersonal psychoanalysis and object relations, as developed within contemporary British theory. But, under the seminal work of the late Stephen A. Mitchell, the term *relational psychoanalysis* grew and began to accrue to itself many other influences and developments. Various tributaries—interpersonal psychoanalysis, object relations theory, self psychology, empirical infancy research, feminism, queer theory, sociocultural studies and elements of contemporary Freudian and Kleinian thought—flow into this tradition, which understands relational configurations between self and others, both real and fantasied, as the primary subject of psychoanalytic investigation.

We refer to the relational tradition, rather than to a relational school, to highlight that we are identifying a trend, a tendency within contemporary psychoanalysis, not a more formally organized or coherent school or system of beliefs. Our use of the term *relational* signifies a dimension of theory and practice that has become salient across the wide spectrum of contemporary psychoanalysis. Now under the editorial supervision of Adrienne Harris and Eyal Rozmarin, the Relational Perspectives Book Series originated in 1990 under the editorial eye of the late Stephen A. Mitchell. Mitchell was the most prolific and influential of the originators of the relational tradition. Committed to dialogue among psychoanalysts, he abhorred the authoritarianism that dictated adherence to a rigid set of beliefs or technical restrictions. He championed open discussion, comparative and integrative approaches, and promoted new voices across the generations. Mitchell was later joined by the late Lewis Aron, also a visionary and influential writer, teacher and leading thinker in relational psychoanalysis.

Included in the Relational Perspectives Book Series are authors and works that come from within the relational tradition, those that extend and develop that tradition, and works that critique relational approaches or compare and contrast them with alternative points of view. The series includes our most distinguished senior psychoanalysts, along with younger contributors who bring fresh vision. Our aim is to enable a deepening of relational thinking while reaching across disciplinary and social boundaries in order to foster an inclusive and international literature.

Note

1 Greenberg, J. & Mitchell, S. (1983). *Object relations in psychoanalytic theory.* Cambridge, MA: Harvard University Press.

A full list of titles in this series is available at https://www.routledge.com/Relational-Perspectives-Book-Series/book-series/LEARPBS.

Psychoanalytic Practices and Russia's War Against Ukraine

Reflections and Clinical Observations

Edited by Mariana Velykodna,
Oksana Yakushko, and
Adrienne Harris

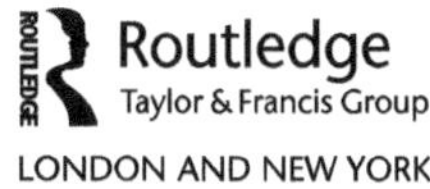

LONDON AND NEW YORK

Designed cover image: Getty Images © TexBr

First published 2026
by Routledge
4 Park Square, Milton Park, Abingdon, Oxon OX14 4RN

and by Routledge
605 Third Avenue, New York, NY 10158

Routledge is an imprint of the Taylor & Francis Group, an informa business

British Library Cataloguing-in-Publication Data
A catalogue record for this book is available from the British Library

ISBN: 978-1-032-66024-0 (hbk)
ISBN: 978-1-032-66023-3 (pbk)
ISBN: 978-1-032-66025-7 (ebk)

DOI: 10.4324/9781032660257

Typeset in Times New Roman
by KnowledgeWorks Global Ltd.

Contents

List of Contributors

Oksana Arshevska-Guerin, M.Sc. in clinical psychology, is a EuroPsy-registered psychologist, a psychodynamic psychotherapist, a lecturer of Psychology Department at Ukraine Sigmund Freud University (Ukraine), and a member of the Psychoanalytic Psychology and Psychotherapy Division of the National Psychological Association of Ukraine.

Yelyzaveta Davoian, Ph.D. in psychology, M.Sc. in psychology, is a EuroPsy-registered psychologist, Head of the Practical Psychology Department at the State University of Economics and Technologies (Ukraine), and a member of the Psychoanalytic Psychology and Psychotherapy Division of the National Psychological Association of Ukraine.

Valeriy Dorozhkin, Sc.D. in psychology, M.Sc. in psychology, is a EuroPsy-registered psychologist, psychoanalytic psychotherapist, certified Balint groups leader, Professor of Theoretical and Practical Psychology Department at the Lviv Polytechnic National University (Ukraine), and Head of the Psychoanalytic Psychology and Psychotherapy Division of the National Psychological Association of Ukraine.

Adrienne Harris, Ph.D., is a faculty and supervisor in the New York University Postdoctoral Program in Psychotherapy and Psychoanalysis, Faculty and Training analyst at the Psychoanalytic Institute of Northern California, and serves on Editorial Boards of several psychoanalytic journals.

Oleh Khrystenko, M.Sc. in clinical psychology, is a psychoanalytic practitioner in private practice (France), a lecturer of psychoanalytic disciplines at the Academy of Social Sciences and Tourism (Ukraine), and a member of the Psychoanalytic Psychology and Psychotherapy Division of the National Psychological Association of Ukraine.

Nina Kokoilo, M.Sc. in clinical psychology, is a certificated specialist of the European Confederation of Psychoanalytic Psychotherapies, a training analyst of the Ukrainian Association for Psychoanalysis, and a member of the Psychoanalytic Psychology and Psychotherapy Division of the National Psychological Association of Ukraine.

Daria Kyrylova, M.Sc. in psychology, is a psychoanalytically oriented psychologist, a EuroPsy-registered psychologist, and a member of the Psychoanalytic Psychology and Psychotherapy Division of the National Psychological Association of Ukraine.

Veronika Lukyanova, M.Sc. in clinical psychology, is a postgraduate student in Neuroscience, a psychoanalytically oriented psychologist, and a member of the Psychoanalytic Psychology and Psychotherapy Division of the National Psychological Association of Ukraine.

Alexander Lupis, Ph.D. in psychology, is a licensed clinical psychologist (Washington, DC), a member and co-chair of the International Relations Committee of the Society for Psychoanalysis and Psychoanalytic Psychology (APA Division 39), and Head of International Division of the National Psychological Association of Ukraine.

Volodymyr Mamko, Ph.D. in psychology, M.Sc. in clinical psychology, is a training analyst and supervisor of the European Confederation of Psychoanalytic Psychotherapies, head of the Institute of Professional Supervision, and a member of the Psychoanalytic Psychology and Psychotherapy Division of the National Psychological Association of Ukraine.

Olena Medvedieva, Ph.D. in philosophy, M.Sc. in clinical psychology, is a psychoanalytic psychotherapist certified by the European Confederation of Psychoanalytic Psychotherapies, a lecturer of psychoanalytic disciplines at the Academy of Social Sciences and Tourism (Ukraine), and a member of the Psychoanalytic Psychology and Psychotherapy Division of the National Psychological Association of Ukraine.

Zoia Miroshnyk, Sc.D. in psychology, is a professor of the Practical Psychology Department at Kryvyi Rih State Pedagogical University (Ukraine) and a member of the Psychoanalytic Psychology and Psychotherapy Division of the National Psychological Association of Ukraine.

Natalia Nalyvaiko, M.Sc. in clinical psychology, is a training analyst and supervisor of the European Confederation of Psychoanalytic

Psychotherapies, and Head of International Relations Committee of the Psychoanalytic Psychology and Psychotherapy Division of the National Psychological Association of Ukraine.

Olena Osypenko, M.Sc. in emergency and crisis psychology, is a training analyst of the Institute of Professional Supervision, a psychoanalyst in private practice (Ukraine), and a member of the Psychoanalytic Psychology and Psychotherapy Division of the National Psychological Association of Ukraine.

Olga Pavlovska, M.Sc. in clinical psychology, is a training analyst of the European Confederation of Psychoanalytic Psychotherapies, a supervisor certified by the Ukrainian Association for Psychoanalysis, a lecturer of the Psychoanalytic Psychotherapy Department at Ukraine Sigmund Freud University (Ukraine), and a member of the Psychoanalytic Psychology and Psychotherapy Division of the National Psychological Association of Ukraine.

Ruslana Rudenko, M.Sc. in psychology, is a training analyst and supervisor of the Odesa Psychoanalytic Society, the Delegate from Ukraine at the Board of the European Federation of Psychoanalytic Psychotherapies, and a member of the Psychoanalytic Psychology and Psychotherapy Division of the National Psychological Association of Ukraine.

Olena Slobodianiuk, M.Sc. in psychology, is a training analyst of the Institute of Professional Supervision, a psychoanalyst in private practice (Ukraine), and a member of the Psychoanalytic Psychology and Psychotherapy Division of the National Psychological Association of Ukraine.

Marianna Tkalych, Sc.D. in psychology, M.Sc. in psychology, is a professor of the Department of Psychology at Zaporizhzhia National University (Ukraine), a professor of the Department of Theoretical and Practical Psychology at Lviv Polytechnic National University (Ukraine), a CEO of the Research Laboratory "Rating Lab", a EuroPsy-registered psychologist, a member of Psychoanalytic Psychology and Psychotherapy Division of the National Psychological Association (Ukraine).

Sergii Ugrium, M.Sc. in psychology, M.Sc. in psychoanalysis, is a EuroPsy-registered psychologist, a psychoanalytic practitioner in private practice, a certified EuroPsy psychologist, a researcher, and a member of the Psychoanalytic Psychology and Psychotherapy Division of the

National Psychological Association of Ukraine (NPA), and works on the NPA's psychological hotline.

Mariana Velykodna, Ph.D. in psychology, M.Sc. in clinical psychology, a EuroPsy-registered psychologist, psychoanalytic psychotherapist certified by the European Confederation of Psychoanalytic Psychotherapies, an associate professor and Head of Psychoanalytic Psychotherapy Department at Ukraine Sigmund Freud University (Ukraine), an associate professor of Practical Psychology Department at Kryvyi Rih State Pedagogical University (Ukraine), a member of Psychoanalytic Psychology and Psychotherapy Division of the National Psychological Association (Ukraine).

Yuliia Vizniuk, Ph.D. in psychology, is a training analyst of the Institute of Professional Supervision, a psychoanalyst in private practice (Ukraine), a lecturer of the Department of General Social and Behavioral Sciences at Volyn Institute of Interregional Academy of Personnel Management, and a member of the Psychoanalytic Psychology and Psychotherapy Division of the National Psychological Association of Ukraine.

Oksana Yakushko, Ph.D., is a licensed psychologist, psychoanalyst, and Ukrainian immigrant. She is a faculty at the George Washington University and a psychoanalytic practitioner in California and Washington, DC. Her scholarship focuses on the histories of psychoanalysis. Since the start of the recent Russian invasion, she has been involved in varied ways to support Ukraine and Ukrainians.

Elina Yevlanova, Ph.D. in psychology, M.Sc. in clinical psychology, is a training analyst of the Institute of Professional Supervision, a psychoanalyst in private practice (Ukraine), a lecturer of the Psychology Department at Ukraine Sigmund Freud University (Ukraine), and a member of the Psychoanalytic Psychology and Psychotherapy Division of the National Psychological Association of Ukraine.

On Psychoanalysts' Avoidance of Knowing More About Wars

Introduction

Mariana Velykodna, Oksana Yakushko, and Adrienne Harris

Typically, the Introduction to a psychoanalytic book offers its readers the context in which the book was written, introduces the gaps in the literature, that the book addressed, and briefly presents key points of each chapter. However, in opening this book, we wanted to envision the Introduction as a counter-point to what occurs outside of such professional efforts. The typical Introduction would demand us to "forget" that we are introducing content—the war—which tends to be avoided, denied, and minimized. Such avoidance is widespread even in the case of psychoanalysis, even while the field claims to offer expertise on defensive patterns in psychic life. In order to situate this book and frame this introductory effort, we begin by turning to some evidentiary material.

One way to ascertain whether the topic of war enters the psychoanalytic zeitgeist is via tracing the evidence in published psychoanalytic materials as well as (available today) who cites or even who reads (downloads) this material. In searches such as PsychInfo, which includes a wider range of psychoanalytic material, it is evident that psychoanalytic contributions were offered, discussed and often critiqued in relation to psychoanalytic responses to psychic origins of war (i.e., aggression, death drive, group defenses) as well as responses to war neuroses and war psychosis. Psychoanalysis, especially Freud's psychoanalytic theorizing, was routinely attacked from 1920 through the 1940s for its supposedly pessimistic insistence that removing social and economic conditions for war or conditioning everyone to be a "pacifist" would work to eliminate wars altogether. However, a review of who reads or cites these materials shows little evidence of psychoanalytic works or their critiques being read or cited. Moreover, certain key psychoanalytic events and contributions, such as the 1918 International Congress of Psychoanalysis, which was in its entirety dedicated to war and working

DOI: 10.4324/9781032660257-1

with war impact, have somehow been transformed into a psychoanalytic contribution to the importance of socialist transformations, which are never mentioned in the congress itself nor in related writings (summary of the Congress and its related events can be found in Ferenczi, 1922).

A more targeted psychoanalytic collection of scholarship specifically focused on access exclusively to psychoanalytic materials, is found in the PEP-web database. A search conducted through the electronic psychoanalytic library PEP-web in May 2024, using search terms such as "war," "wars," and "wartime" in the titles of published papers revealed that only a few of these works were viewed, and even fewer cited (Table 0.1). It looks especially remarkable compared to uses of the term "trauma" which is the leading topic of psychoanalytic works published from 1900 to 2019, having progressively increased its appearance since the 1940s in the post-World War II period (Knafo et al., 2022). Notably, prior to the increase in the use of the word "trauma," related terms such as shell shock, war neuroses, and war psychoses were utilized in both psychoanalytic and related scholarship (Koteska, 2019, 2020). However, progressively the focus on war itself in psychoanalytic literature has been diminished or erased. Outside of the impact of the Holocaust trauma, psychoanalytic histories, and writings minimize or erase the context of war. For example, German

Table 0.1 Viewed and Cited Papers Devoted to War Topics Deposed at PEP-web (Searched on May 19, 2024; PEP-web, 2024)

Variable	*War*	*Wars*	*Wartime*
View Count			
0–9 views (number of papers)	371	12	20
10–19 views (number of papers)	46	1	2
20–29 views (number of papers)	17	2	—
30–39 views (number of papers)	6	—	—
70–1579 views (number of papers)	4	—	—
Citation Count			
0 citations (number of papers)	380	11	18
1–5 citations (number of papers)	61	4	4
6–9 citations (number of papers)	2	—	—
10–25 citations (number of papers)	1	—	—
Number of papers in Total	444	15	22

psychoanalytic contribution to conversations about "Mourning and Melancholia" by Freud, Ferenczi, and Abraham between 1915 and 1918 by May (2019) in the *International Journal of Psychoanalysis* mentions war only as an impediment for these individuals to get together rather than exchange correspondence, and concludes that despite the "morally despicable actions" during the "World War II" and the "Holocaust," the "fundamental rule of psychoanalysis," apparent to the author, is found in a "temporary suspension of moral judgment" (p. 94). Such a stunning conclusion on the contributions and discussions of three founders of psychoanalysis, all of whom not only were working amidst war but actively engaged in its efforts and its aftermath (e.g., Ferenczi was an active military psychiatrist, conducting "equine psychoanalysis" between military action), is a kind of "confusion of tongues," about which Ferenczi will come to write later.

Titles of contributions reveal a lot, in our view. As noted above, conducting a search of titles on the PEP-web revealed the following patterns in not just the uses of these terms by psychoanalytic authors (not many) but especially in how many times these contributions were viewed or cited within the digital archive.

Thus, of 444 contributions in total on the PEP-web, they are rarely viewed and rarely cited. Naming the war, it seems, is just as difficult as being open to witness it. This contribution, as we stress, is written by individuals who do not and cannot avoid the context of the war. They are living and working with patients, even as this Introduction is written, under a full-scale violent military invasion, under continued threat of death, violence, torture, and destruction of their homes. Wars have been continuously fought throughout the last and this century. While many in contemporary US based psychoanalysis equate wars with American imperialism and capitalism (i.e., reducing wars in Korea, Vietnam, and Afghanistan to these categories exclusively), it is not the war or war context per se they are interested in. Moreover, the narcissistic self-focus on the wrongness of all American military actions tends to ignore wars and military violence worldwide, especially those perpetuated continuously by the Russian Federation in territories it colonized (e.g., Chechnya), it seeks to colonize (e.g., Georgia, Moldova, Ukraine), or where it seeks to gain colonial influence via its violent mercenary military actions (e.g., Syria, Mali). Wars, we insist, if present at all, are either backdrop for social self-critiques or, far more commonly, a context erased. In defended, almost negatively hallucinatory representations, wars, past and present, are either entirely absent or become merely "bad" decorative backgrounds that can be ignored. Wars, and not just war trauma, must be witnessed, theorized, and studied in psychoanalysis. This book offers such contributions to the field.

Responses to War

As we noted, it appears that the psychoanalytic community, in general, is far more open to dealing with war effects: trauma (including its transgenerational legacies—see a recent study by Knafo, 2004; Lupis et al., 2023), losses (Pavlovska, 2023), or war-forced migration issues (Beltsiou, 2016). Psychoanalytic societies worldwide offer war victims (i.e., war refugees) different mental health initiatives, typically collapsing their care together with all other "people in need." During wars scholarships for colleagues from war-affected countries and, especially, seminars, pieces of training, and certificates usually on how to "work with trauma" is another response. Very few contributions have been made to contemporary psychoanalytically informed interventions for people in crises that were directly caused by wars (e.g., Leuzinger-Bohleber et al., 2016). However, exploring the origins of war as an ongoing human phenomenon, especially by not collapsing all "wars" (i.e., civil, military interventions, responses to genocides) but rather focusing on each specific war with its historic and present-day context, is rare. Psychoanalysts do not appear focused on socio-psychological and psychic conditions in which the production of such wars occur, or in the social dissemination, processing, and termination of wars. Among exceptions, in our view, are works by scholars that seek to focus on this topic today (e.g., Alderdice, 2022, 2024; Lupis, 2024; Ramzy, 2022; Wood, 2024).

Moreover, we have observed that psychoanalytic scholars who attempt to theorize about wars and political leaders who launch them, often face criticism that psychoanalysts should not become involved in such analyses and should maintain neutrality (e.g., Papazian, 2022). Another pattern is to remind such scholars that they must recognize the limits of their methods in exploring wars and their leaders (e.g., García-García, 2024). In addition, the Kremlin-based justification that its war against Ukraine was merely a pre-emptive self-defensive war against the ubiquitous "West," psychoanalytic scholars, are used to silence efforts to discuss the Russian aggression and its perpetrators. For instance, D'Agostino (2022), the scholarly leader and editor of psychoanalytically based psychohistory organizations, responded to one such effort by Ihanus and Beisel by stating that "by putting

Vladimir Putin on the couch and omitting objective security threats to which the Russian leader apparently responded, these psychohistorians demonize Putin and implicitly exonerate the U.S. and NATO for their roles in the conflict" (p. 82). D'Agostino is far from alone among psychoanalytically informed scholars and psychoanalysts outside of Ukraine whose ahistoric and deliberately obfuscating response denies reality. In many ways, such response to dictatorial violent wars by "progressive" presenting scholars is not new: O'Neill (2022) and many others documented how far justifications of both Stalin's violence, as well as for Hitler during the over two years of World War II of Stalin-Hitler pact and joint invasion, extended among American intellectuals and cultural leaders. In repeated public pronouncements by varied progressive and anti-war intellectuals of that era in the United States, both Stalin and Hitler were "provoked" and were merely "defending" themselves against "imperialist Britain and France." George Orwell's essays during 1930s and 1940s were dedicated in large part to naming and understanding this same pattern among the British and European intellectuals, who venerated violent aggressive regimes of Hitler and Stalin as somehow "peaceful" and merely responding to "threats." Similar narratives and explanations abound in relation to the new Russian invasion of Ukraine in 2022, regardless of available histories, information, or even self-articulated goals in this war by Putin and the Russian Federation representatives.

Numerous Ukraine-based psychoanalytic professionals began to highlight that they face these and other symptomatic responses from the international psychodynamic audiences. In addition to both unawareness of history and unwillingness to know it, global psychoanalytic communities have been experienced by Ukrainian psychoanalysts as tending to deny and minimize the brutality of this war or "explaining" it concepts designed to subvert the reality, which is experienced as violent by Ukrainians (e.g., Garmish, 2024; Romanov, 2023; Velykodna, 2024). In many ways, this book is an invitation to witness, listen, learn, and seek to understand this war (and wars) from psychoanalytically based clinicians who are living and working amidst it, and all of whom have lived and worked with the impact of long-standing history of Russia's imperial colonial aggression against Ukraine and Ukrainians. Using the term of the book by leading contemporary historian Snyder (2010), Ukraine has been the "bloodlands," both in relation to continued Russian to violently occupy and control it as well as how much the global community has been willing to use Ukraine for negotiation of its own guilt, politics, denial, projection, and economic gain. In this book, the readers are invited to engage with the experiences of war—via individual psychoanalytic sessions, crisis lines, groups on de-occupied territories, family work, supervision, refugees, and others—through direct experiences and analysis by Ukrainians themselves.

In our view, the most important contribution of this book is not in offering cutting-edge interdisciplinary critiques. We do not analyze the war through the lens of modern consumer society (White, 2022) or neo-liberation policies (Hollander, 2023), which are concerns of American audiences based on their socio-political histories. This contribution is designed to describe psychoanalytic work and life during the war by individuals directly impacted by it. In our view, a similar effort was made at the fifth International Psychoanalytic Congress in Budapest in 1918, which was devoted entirely to World War I and war-based impact (e.g., shell shock, war neuroses, war psychoses), Freud, Ferenczi, Abraham, Jones, and other psychoanalysts took the Congress as an opportunity to speak directly to European military and government authorities. All of the above-mentioned psychoanalytic pioneers stressed that they directly worked and lived these war experiences (i.e., on the war front lines, in military hospitals, or in practices dedicated to working with war wounded). They discussed the war effects they observed and critiqued extant methods of treatment (e.g., electric shock, medication, and auto-suggestion as treatment modalities). They offered innovative paths toward creating forms of psychotherapy that addressed the war and postwar symptoms, documenting that their work demonstrated superiority to then-common psychiatric treatments (Muñoz & Correia, 2022).

Notably, in the introduction to the congress proceedings, which was published a few years after it took place, Freud (1921) stressed that as soon as World War I officially ended, the interest in the topic of war and treating its impact, including among government representatives, almost entirely stopped. Recent historical investigations reveal that in contrast to the realities that war-based trauma care predominated all medical and mental health-related fields during the early 20th century in Europe, the postwar period appeared to be marked by nearly immediate efforts to forget war experiences. Such defensive forgetting, denial, repression, and disassociation are certainly what have become linked to long-term and generational traumatic legacies (Davoine, 2010) as well as to other patterns of dissociation related to all types of trauma in general (Harris, 2010). This dissociation, including among analysts, had further effects.

According to Hollander's (2023) interview with Mimi Langer, the psychoanalytic community in Vienna denied it. At the start of World War II, the psychoanalytic community tended to deny its threat. Langer was an analyst from Argentina, who began her psychoanalytic training at Vienna Psychoanalytic Institute in 1935, just as fascism spread through Europe. She remembered her astonishment at how the threat of war, growing every year, was minimally discussed in psychoanalytic circles and that the psychoanalytic community believed itself to be invulnerable to Nazism (Hollander, 2023). Recent histories with a focus on this era show that Freud was among those who minimized the potential threats and delayed escaping, even at the grave risk of violence and death (Nagorski, 2022). Psychoanalytic historians provide evidence that psychoanalysts were involved not only as those who fight the war-related effects in populations but also who supported or minimized the war violence (e.g., Yakushko, 2023). Certainly, denying war threats and avoiding acknowledging its cruelty was at times covered by ideological frameworks (as discussed above in relation to the promotion of Bolshevism but also to adherence to Social Darwinism and eugenics).

These pieces of historical and recent evidence raise questions about these powerful forces, operating behind the processes of denial, avoidance, and forgetting mass cruelty and violence, especially for those not living amidst wars or anticipating wars to be brought to them (i.e., wars at times only entered into thinking when personal threat from nuclear weaponry was acknowledged). Certainly, we cannot address this issue fully in this brief introduction. We do believe that there has been insufficient attention to this and other topics related to war in psychoanalytic theorizing and research. We are aware of few such efforts. For example, defensive avoidance of discussing wars has been analyzed as a form of repudiated self-reflection in order to mitigate guilt among perpetrators of war crimes and their family members (Mitscherlich & Mitscherlich, 1975). Clinicians who worked with war trauma experienced by war victims and war witnesses also contributed to understanding how highly traumatized people elect the avoidance of talking about wars because of numerous obstacles, especially a lack of social recognition of their experience by others (Bohleber, 2007). However, we are not aware of psychoanalytic theorizing about the reasons for the avoidance of knowing, listening, and talking about wars among people who do not have direct war-related personal history. Notably, Freud's theories about the fear of annihilation and the uncanny, Winnicott's work on primitive anxieties and relevant agonies, or challenges with capacities toward recognition of cruelty (Akhtar, 2024) may contribute to unconscious processes evoked by wars among those who do not have to live through them. Another theoretical development is to examine the specific war modes of psychic functioning, as suggested by one of the book's authors Velykodna (2024). The totalitarian state of mind is possibly another psychic pattern that leads individuals to deny, minimize, or purposefully obfuscate the realities of war (Semkiv, 2024). These and other defensive strategies in relation to engaging with the topic of war and its impact must be further examined, considering that war are an ongoing living reality for individuals worldwide. In reading this book, we hope that the reader engages in self-reflection and self-analysis in relation to their own openness or resistance to being with the realities of war.

Book Outline

This book is a collection of writings by Ukrainian psychoanalysts and psychoanalytically informed practitioners who have been conducting their work under conditions of Russian aggression against Ukraine. As noted above, the world wars (both World War I and II, and other global conflicts) have been instrumental in shaping psychoanalysis as a discipline, especially its theories of trauma (Ferenczi, 1922; Freud, 1920; Koteska, 2019, 2020; Midgley, 2007; Reeves, 2004). Moreover, psychoanalysts, starting with Freud (1921) and Ferenczi, Abraham, Jones, and others (1922), stressed that psychoanalytic forms of care were vitally important for helping address brutal conditions of wars and their impact not only on children and adults but also on analysts themselves. This contribution by Ukrainian psychoanalysts similarly carries such weight in its broad spectrum of contributions by Ukrainian analysts. In addition to describing processes and experiences of working and theorizing by psychoanalytic clinicians under conditions of ongoing violent war, this contribution also highlights many other aspects, including the impact of multigenerational trauma, severe psychopathology, and phenomenological subjective realities of being objectified as a subhuman, fantasies, and language on people who survive such aggression. Ethical struggles, working under continued conditions of death, forced terminations, and significant losses are discussed via cases and observations. The psychoanalysts in this contribution also discuss their work with vulnerable and diverse cultural groups, including children and adolescents, war refugees, individuals in severe physical and psychological crises, and Ukrainian Jews. Contributions also introduce the readers to remarkable clinical innovations by Ukrainian psychoanalysts in these conditions: war-time daily supervision groups, relational peer-led groups, and collaborative interdisciplinary organizations. Lastly, this contribution also includes voices of Ukrainian psychoanalysts who work within the international psychoanalytic community and with Ukrainian diaspora members in the United States.

Like the ongoing war, the volume is not organized in before and after, or who might be the most impacted. The war is a totalizing atrocity against human and non-human beings, against society and its living culture, against life itself. The war also requires responses that cannot be predicted or even imagined in non-war times. The book begins with a chapter by Nalyvaiko, who articulates the connection between numerous generational forms of trauma Ukrainians experienced, including in her family, and the present-day war. Dorozhkin's contribution focuses on the remarkable responses to war, starting with the earliest days of a brutal full-scale invasion, in which psychoanalytic clinicians and other colleagues organized as a containing group space for each other as well as a method for mobilizing in responding in some of the most vulnerable communities. In his chapter, the documented work in offering individual and group therapeutic interventions to individuals from de-occupied territories, where people and entire communities were tortured (and not metaphorically), witnessed horrific brutality (gang rapes, executions, targeted destruction), and where Russian troops used systematic efforts of ripping all social ties and fabrics (e.g., lies about political reality or about neighbors turning them in). Both the witnesses of these aspects of war and the response are detailed and theorized about, using both documented evidence and narratives. Vizniuk and Yevlanova focus on examining cases that show how Oedipal development and conflicts interact with the context of war, providing valuable theoretical contributions both understanding the psychic war impact as well as intricacies of the individual Oedipal patterns under violent circumstances. Using a Lacanian-based framework, Medvedieva focuses on what is speech during the war, especially how the silence, the tears, and the voice reflect the real, both as the Symbolic and the Imaginary, in working with people whose lives Russian aggression torn apart.

Pavlovska and Kokoilo document their work and theorize on what occurs for individuals who have non-neurotic (i.e., psychotic) psychic organization. Understanding how the external destructive context interacts with the already compromised internally destructive psychic world in such a situation offers important insights into both the clinical understanding of non-neurotic patients (who can face war and other externally violent events) as well as the evocative power of violence on complex psychic lives. Considering work with these and other patients (and non-patients), also requires the struggle with the notion of ethics in working during the war. Psychoanalytic ethics, such as notions of analytic neutrality and abstinence and self-disclosure, are challenged and upturned in war times. General clinical practice ethics in relation to dual roles, confidentiality, competence to practice, self-care, and more become practical impossibilities while still requiring attention. Lastly, the ethics of continuing work with individuals who represent the aggressor-state is another war-based ethical consideration, which is discussed by Arshevska-Guérin, Nalyvaiko, and Velykodna in their chapter on ethics. In a related piece, Khrystenko documents and analyzes the impact of war on the psychoanalytic treatment process, focusing on the intense effects and affects of war in the psychic container of analytic work. Velykodna and Knafo further discussed the issues related to termination during the war, considering the levels of practical therapeutic aspects of endings as well as their psychic meanings in transference-countertransference space.

In a chapter with a focus on distinct defensive patterns in transference among Ukrainian war refugees to other countries, Yevlanova highlights the psychic defenses and phantasies among individuals who left Ukraine in search of safety. Slobodianiuk and Osypenko focus on psychoanalytic group engagement with another distinct Ukrainian community facing the war—the Ukrainian Jewish community—noting how the generational impact of both the Holocaust and Soviet-based violence toward Jewish identity in Ukraine shapes the community survival and community function during the war.

In addition to group work in communities, presented in the above chapters (e.g., Dorozhkin, Slobodianiuk, and Osypenko), the Ukrainian psychoanalytic community had to face other adaptations to therapeutic practice during the war. One of such adaptations is the vital necessity of mental health crisis lines, considering that individuals under constant direct threat of violence and destruction, often can seek out singular brief links to help from others. Ugrium discusses what it means to work psychoanalytically via a mental health crisis line. We are not aware of any other similar psychoanalytic contributions, and Ugrium's description of how one-time crisis line contact can hold the focus of psychoanalytic values of containment, mentalization, and stress on possibilities for crisis line callers' libidinal life investment, offers a distinct and remarkable view of psychoanalytic' possibilities during the war. Davoian, Kyrylova, and Miroshnyk's chapter further described the challenges of working with children and their parents during the war. Parents, whose parental psychic lives might already be marked by compromised defensive patterns, are shown to struggle in psychically containing their children's experience of war. This contribution is important in its illustration of ways in which the psychic context of war shapes psychic parental processes and (certainly) child development.

Equally important is the process offered in psychoanalytic supervision for analysts and clinicians who continue working with the war's "front lines" in their offices or in public spaces via groups. Mamko's work illustrates the process of supervision during the war, including cases in which supervision dynamics and experiences highlight the many vicissitudes of such work. Another chapter, focused on supervision, describes the distinct collaborative and peer-based Intervision supervisory development, development and process of which is described by Lukyanova and Rudenko. Possibilities of such peer-supervisory spaces to contain therapists' own experience of war terror are illustrated in their contribution.

The last chapter in this book focuses on psychoanalytic developments in relation to war in Ukraine outside of Ukraine's borders. Lupis, Tkalych, and Velykodna focus on international developments, involvement, and relations between Ukrainian and global psychoanalytic communities during the first two years since full-scale Russian invasion of Ukraine. The chapter focuses on various efforts to support the psychoanalytic Ukrainian community in responding to the war crisis, supporting continued access to psychoanalytic care, increasing the representation of Ukrainian psychoanalytic voices in global psychoanalytic spaces, and envisioning the future of Ukrainian psychoanalysis.

Conclusion

At the time of writing this book, there has been no solution to Russian aggression against Ukraine. International authorities, designed to supposedly address such global atrocities and to ensure justice, have predominately failed. Russia continues its war efforts with unmitigated freedom in the use of all the internationally banned methods, processes, weapons, or practices (e.g., bombings, kidnapping, torture, rape, attacks on civilian infrastructure, destruction of cultural heritage, targeted bombings of hospitals and schools, uses of nuclear threat and more). The voices, even at the start of the full-scale invasion, that described Russia as peace-keeping, threated, self-protective, and liberatory, have become even more prominent, including in psychoanalysis, with their continued ahistoric and politically narcissistic analyses (e.g., "this war is all about our guilt" or "we have done something like Russia so have no right to respond"). Numerous other false, defensive, obfuscating and at times patently propagandist positions veil this war and its impacts. Behind the smoke screens, erected by distance and distancing, Ukrainian psychoanalysts have been working while facing this war. This book is an invitation to be with them—to witness, to mentalize, and to integrate an understanding of war into our psychoanalytic (or other) frameworks of understanding psychological responses to war. This book in many ways is a counter-point to what Velykodna (2023) described as the psychic mode of war, which often operates to defend people and groups against the very real lived realities of war.

There has been no conclusion to this war. Possibly, wars cannot have a conclusion, considering their horrific lasting, and generational impact on people who were intentionally targeted and dehumanized (e.g., they asked for it). This book is a contribution to un-silencing the work on war through contributions by Ukrainian psychoanalysts and psychoanalytically informed clinicians for whom this war remains a deafening presence.

References

Akhtar, S. (2024). On human cruelty. *International Journal of Applied Psychoanalytic Studies*, 21(2), e1864.

Alderdice, J. (2022). Can a focus on the importance of relationships help us address the pandemic of violence? *The International Journal of Forensic Psychotherapy*, 4(2), 192–207.

Alderdice, J. L. (2024). New insights into the psychology of individuals and large groups in a world of changing conflicts. *International Political Science Review*, 45(1), 94–105.

Beltsiou, J. (2016). *Immigration in psychoanalysis*. London: Routledge.

Bohleber, W. (2007). Remembrance, trauma and collective memory: The battle for memory in psychoanalysis. *The International Journal of Psychoanalysis*, 88(2), 329–352. https://doi.org/10.1516/V5H5-8351-7636-7878

Davoine, F. (2010). Casus belli. In A. Harris, S. Botticelli (Eds.). *First do no harm*. New York: Taylor and Francis.

D'Agostino, B. (2022). Psychohistory, Ideology, and Ukraine: A Reply to Juhani Ihanus and David Beisel. *The Journal of Psychohistory*, 50, 2.

Ferenczi, S. (1922). *Psychoanalysis and the war neuroses*. New York: G.E. Stechert.

Freud, S. (1920). Beyond the pleasure principle. In J. Strachey (Ed.). *The standard edition of the complete psychological works of Sigmund Freud, Vol. XVIII (1720–1922): Beyond the Pleasure Principle, Group Psychology and Other Works, 1–64*. London: Hogarth Press.

Freud, S. (1921). Introduction. In S. Ferenci, K. Abraham, E. Simmel, E. Jones (Eds.). *Psycho-analysis and the war neuroses* (pp. 7–14). M.V.: New York: G.E. Stechert.

García-García, J. (2024). The war of Vladimir. Nationalism, narcissism, and childhood battles. *Journal of Nationalism, Memory & Language Politics*. https://doi.org/10.2478/jnmlp-2024-0001

Garmish, P. (2024). A letter from the front: A message from a psychoanalyst defending Ukraine from the Russian invasion. *Psychoanalytic Inquiry*, 45(4), 393–403. https://doi.org/10.1080/07351690.2024.2355192

Harris, A. (2010). Ferenczi's work on war neuroses. *Psychoanalytic Perspectives*, 7(1), 183–190. https://doi.org/10.1080/1551806X.2010.10473082

Hollander, N.C. (2023). *Uprooted minds. A social psychoanalysis for precarious times*. 2nd ed. New York: Routledge.

Knafo, D. (Ed.). (2004). *Living with terror, working with trauma: A clinician's handbook*. USA: Jason Aronson.

Knafo, D., Oxholm, B. & Snyder, S. A. (2022). In our own words: Key terms and trends in psychoanalytic history. *American Journal of Psychoanalysis*, 82, 512–547. https://doi.org/10.1057/s11231-022-09376-5

Koteska, J. (2019). Freud on the First World War (Part 1). Researcher. *European Journal of Humanities & Social Sciences*. 4(2), 53–68.

Koteska, J. (2020). Freud on the First World War (Part 2). *Researcher. European Journal of Humanities & Social Sciences*. 1(3), 45–60.

Leuzinger-Bohleber, M., Rickmeyer, C., Tahiri, M., Hettich, N., & Fischmann, T. (2016). What can psychoanalysis contribute to the current refugee crisis? *The International Journal of Psychoanalysis*, 97(4), 1077–1093. https://doi.org/10.1111/1745-8315.12542

Lupis, A. (2024). Leadership analysis in international affairs: A psychodynamic perspective. *Ukrainian Psychoanalytic Journal*, 2(1), 108–117. https://doi.org/10.32782/upj/2024-1-12

Lupis, A., Meehan, K., Wong, P., Haden, S., & Kuterovac Jagodić, G. (2023). Intergenerational transmission of trauma in Croatia: Relational anger & guilt in children of combat veterans. *Ukrainian Psychoanalytic Journal*, 1(1), 36–46. https://doi.org/10.32782/upj/2023-1-7

Midgley, N. (2007). Anna Freud: The Hampstead War Nurseries and the role of the direct observation of children for psychoanalysis. *The International Journal of Psychoanalysis*, 88(4), 939–959.

Mitscherlich, A., Mitscherlich, M. (1975). *The inability to mourn: Principles of collective behaviour*. New York: Grove.

Muñoz, P., & Correia, S. (2022). The great war and the fifth international psychoanalytic congress in Budapest: Psychoanalysis in the 1910s. Historia Crítica, (84), 3–27. https://doi.org/10.7440/histcrit84.2022.01

O'Neill, D. (2022). Salvatore D'Urso 1927–2022. *The Queensland Journal of Labour History*, (35), 79–92. https://search.informit.org/doi/10.3316/informit.726121221902710

Nagorski, A. (2022). Saving Freud: A Life in Vienna and an Escape to Freedom in London. Icon Books.

Papazian, B. (2022). Le négatif de la séduction de masse lors de l'invasion russe en Ukraine. Revue Belge de Psychanalyse, (2), 117–129.

Pavlovska, O. (2023). Psychoanalytic work with losses during the war: The Ukrainian experience. *Psychoanalytic Psychology*, 40(4), 251. https://doi.org/10.1037/pap0000479

PEP-web. (2024). Psychoanalytic electronic publishing. https://pep-web.org/ Accessed May 19, 2024.

Ramzy, N. (2022). The existential threat of nuclear war: A psychoanalytic comment. *International Journal of Applied Psychoanalytic Studies*, 19(1), 3–15.

Reeves, C. (2004). On being" intrinsical": A Winnicott enigma. American Imago, 61(4), 427–455.

Romanov, I. (2023). Equation, moralization, and denial. *Psychoanalysis, Culture & Society*, 28(1), 109–115. https://doi.org/10.1057/s41282-022-00339-4

Semkiv, I. (2024). War: Mentalization and totalitarian state of mind. *The Journal of Analytical Psychology*. https://doi.org/10.1111/1468-5922.12987

Snyder, T. (2010). *Bloodlands: Europe Between Hitler and Stalin: Europe Between Hitler and Stalin*. Bodley Head Limited.

Velykodna, M. (2023). A psychoanalyst's experience of working in wartime: On choosing between bad options. *Psychoanalytic Psychology*, 40(4). http://doi.org/10.1037/pap0000480

Velykodna, M. (2024). War and attacks on thinking: Reflections on the psychoanalysts' responses to the 2022 Russian invasion of Ukraine. *Psychoanalytic Inquiry*, 45(4), 340–362. https://doi.org/10.1080/07351690.2024.2355172

White, J. R. (2022). Colonizing the American psyche: Virtue and the problem of consumer capitalism. In *Critical theory and psychoanalysis* (pp. 211–230). New York: Routledge.

Wood, R. (Ed.). (2024). *Psychoanalytic reflections on Vladimir Putin: The cost of malignant leadership*. Abingdon, England: Routledge.

Yakushko, O. (2023). Psychoanalysis and war: Histories of theorizing, resistance and support for war violence. *Ukrainian Psychoanalytic Journal*, 1(1), 14–20. https://doi.org/10.32782/upj/2023-1-3

Chapter 1

In the Nets of Trauma

Ukrainian Case

Natalia Nalyvaiko

> To my father, Victor Ivanenko, an anticolonial doer, from whom I learned that even in the darkness of the totalitarian regime, one is able to resist colonial enslavement.

This big war which Russia started against Ukraine on the 24th of February, as the geographically and politically largest land war in Europe after the Second World War, has become one the most significant humanitarian catastrophes in Europe of the 21st century. However, by implementing this act of aggression, which is recognized by international law as invasion, Russia had in mind a different signifier. Absorbing over centuries Ukrainian territories, imposing the discourse of a joined history, culture, land, insisting on speaking the same language – Russian, abolishing the Ukrainian one, encouraging to fight same enemies and celebrate same victories, pretending to be "a single nation" therefore perceiving Ukraine as an "integral" and "inseparable" part of the Russian territory, a spoiled part of Russia's self, Russia declared it came to rescue. Even more – "Ukraine is, of course, Russia" (Medvedev, 2024a). Russia came to rescue, to defend, to liberate Ukraine… from Ukraine.

Russian ex-president, currently the Deputy Chairman of the Russian Security Council, Dmitriy Medvedev, declared that the existence of Ukraine is a constant pretext for military action by Russia because "Existence of Ukraine is mortally dangerous for Ukrainians. Ukraine must… recognize that the entire territory of Ukraine is the territory of the Russian Federation," — Medvedev (2024b) pronounced recently.

Ukraine, in Russia's perception, just had to be repaired, but in a perversive Orwellian way where the invasion was called liberation; genocide/de-Ukrainification was termed de-Nazification; deportations were named an

DOI: 10.4324/9781032660257-2

adoption. These psychotic and befuddling war slogans, marked by a complete reversal of the meaning, were etched on the bloody flags of the invader and complicated an already complex trauma that exists among Ukrainians.

Therefore, in order to fully understand the experiences of the present, not just this war and its large-scale humanitarian crises, these events, and their impact must be viewed from the perspective of the numerous massive collective traumas – the most essential ones – totalitarian colonial trauma – which have brutally (re)visited upon Ukraine throughout its history. This exploration not only requires an understanding of the specific traumas experienced by the Ukrainian people but also an examination of the mechanisms through which these traumas are transmitted across generations and the ways in which they shape the collective psyche of the nation.

Collective Trauma

Ukraine's history is marked by a series of traumatic events, and Ukrainian people face severe traumatic circumstances, often without being able to process or heal from the previous ones. From generation to generation, Ukrainians face tragic events that often overlap and remain the source of their mass generational collective traumas. They are two world wars, civil wars, artificial famines, violent killings, repressions, numerous mass deportations, cultural oppression, Soviet big terror, the Holocaust, the Chernobyl disaster, and now is a new war (Plokhy, 2023; Snyder, 2010). Because human memory mainly functions in a collective context (Halbwachs, 2020) these events also live in a group's collective memory long after the actual trauma has resolved. These processes often impact the decisions people make, the values they hold, and the way they live.

These events and their consequences have had profound impacts on the collective psyche of its people. Each of them has left deep scars on the national consciousness and unconscious throughout centuries, contributing to a collective trauma that is revisited with each new crisis from generation to generation. The collective trauma of this kind which includes genocide, civil war, slavery, institutional oppression, and totalitarian regimes, thus one which arises from the impact of colonization, has been defined as cultural or historical trauma (Brave Heart & Chase, 2011). It was also termed the intergenerational trauma (Brave Heart & Debruyn, 1998) and the colonial trauma (Evans-Campbell, 2008).

Context of Collective Trauma in Ukraine

Given the context in which Ukraine during centuries was in its relationship with Russia, the Ukrainian collective trauma is considered transgenerational totalitarian colonial trauma. The mixture of these two traumas determined the trajectory of Ukraine's development. Totalitarian trauma is associated with the use of force. In this case, the state is super-powerful, unaccountable, and controls almost every aspect of a person's life. Any manifestation of leadership or subjectivity increases the risk of death. Totalitarianism carries particular transgenerational toxicity because the government uses indoctrination and brainwashing to exercise power and control, and often the difference between victims and perpetrators is unclear, suggested Cherepanova (2020) about the Soviet totalitarian state.

From a psychoanalytic standpoint, transgenerational trauma is understood as a process through which the unresolved traumas of one generation are passed down to subsequent generations, influencing their emotional and psychological development. This collective experience leaves a profound mark on cultural identity and is accompanied by a sense of collective victimhood, Cherepanova (2020) stressed. This transmission can occur through direct communication of traumatic experiences, but it also happens in more subtle ways, such as through behaviors, attitudes, and the emotional climate within families and communities.

Salberg (Grand & Salberg, 2016; Salberg, 2017), examining trauma from a psychoanalytical stance, explained that the violence of trauma fractures someone's experience of being in the world and tears at the fabric of attachment. Ruptures in attachment relationships that occur in trauma become one of the key mechanisms of how it is transmitted to the next generation. The scars from traumas that are inside of people who become parents often affect directly their capacity to be consistent and engaged in their caregiving. Unresolved mourning and persistent states of anxiety, depression, and terror interfere with attaching and trusting new relationships. While many survivors of trauma also transmit resiliency and want to create loving families and communities, more often, trauma survivors carry both resiliency and the scars of trauma. It is the imprint of the dehumanizing aspects of trauma, the violent victimization of one's integrity as a person as well as surviving when others perished that continues to haunt survivors. These ghosts of their past get transmitted and can be seen in successive generations.

The concept of the "crypt," which is quite similar to "ghost," introduced by Nicolas Abraham, offers a useful metaphor for understanding how unspoken and unresolved traumas can haunt subsequent generations (Abrams, 1999). These phantoms represent the secret traumas of ancestors, buried within the family narrative but exerting influence on the descendants. In the Ukrainian context, the collective silence and denial surrounding events like the Holodomor have created such phantoms, leading to a pervasive sense of loss and mourning that permeates the national consciousness.

In her psychoanalytical research on colonial trauma, Lazari (2021) theorized about silence, unspeakable, which is always present in the colonial trauma bears unconscious. She noted that terror, beyond trauma, is a psychic state that doesn't reveal itself in speech and cannot be repressed but seizes physical bodies and, at the same time, in the same indistinguishable impulse, the social body as well. Maintaining silence is a direct effect of the genocide, the way the mothers communicated with their children about the trauma (Bezo & Maggi, 2015). First of all, because it is unbearable to remember, it is repressed into the unconscious, and transmitted through behavior, beliefs, and particular messages.

The leading message of Soviet/Russian totalitarian culture was "keep your head down." It was a kind of "survival messages" (Cherepanov, 2020) indicating that life is dangerous. Survival messages are trauma-related life lessons that are communicated transgenerationally as condensed prescriptions that parents use to instruct their children in order to keep them safe and teach them how to deal with the adversity their parents were exposed to (Cherepanov, 2020). These messages that they pass on to their children and grandchildren are mostly dealing with untrust and communication with the Other, which is always dangerous. They often follow these lines: "Don't trust, don't ask for help – you will be betrayed anyway – you can't change anything." While the messages may have initially helped people stay alive, in the present, they are often irrelevant and may even increase people's interpersonal vulnerability. Thus, the historical collective experience of victimization is becoming a part of cultural identity. This already unconscious incorporated fear manifests itself as reactive formation in the form of avoidance of direct contacts, lies, opportunism, corruption, and procrastination in relation to the Other.

Bar-On et al. (1998), among other scholars, focused on the notion of the "conspiracy of silence," a pattern that would hide past horrors from children and protect parents from painful memories. Silence about the past, however, has a negative impact on parenting and may create an incoherent and lopsided trauma discourse that promotes fear and victimhood and restricts the right to happiness. There were many families who had some kind of mysterious "uncle" who disappeared and was never spoken about. And there were different kinds of silence.

Personal Experience

When I was a child, some things in my environment seemed strange to me. For example, why have I never had grandparents? One, my mother's father, was killed in the war, I knew that. No one knew where the second grandfather had gone; they said he had "disappeared."

Why do you need to eat a lot (grandmother said – just for reserve) and why everything with bread? Why did the grandmother's neighbors whisper that her neighbor Baba Katya ate a child when it was a big hunger, and therefore, she is crazy? What does it mean – she "ate a child"? It was very scary to hear that. Why did Uncle Ivan change his surname from Ukrainian Petrenko to Russian Petrov? Why can't you trust anyone, but you have to check everything? Why do you need to speak Russian and not Ukrainian to please the teacher? Why are there so many mysteries that are not explained? We never knew our grandfather from the father's side. Grandma said that he disappeared in 1935, a year after my father was born, and my father never saw him, of course, and he did not know also where he had gone. But sometimes the grandmother remembered that the grandfather called Stalin a thief and said that collective farms stink. These were the times of Stalinist repressions, and apparently, Grandfather had not disappeared by accident. We never talked about this unspoken secret, and we never solved it. This was a family "crypt."

I think that it was precisely this gap in memory that my father unconsciously tried to fill, devoting his entire life to opposing totalitarianism. Otherwise, why did he choose this dangerous path of otherness and dissidence in a totally controlled country? Like Fanon, who was "the most influential anticolonial thinker" (Jansen & Osterhammel, 2017, p. 164) my father was the greatest anticolonial doer. My husband's father's silence was about his imprisonment in a German concentration camp during the war; my husband's mother's silence was about her sister's death during Holodomor, their uncle's arrest, and imprisonment in a Soviet concentration camp for hiding some grain during the artificial starvation. My husband never learned about it. Once, when he was refused a job in a state institution because he was the nephew of an "enemy of the people," he asked his mother about it. Deaf silence was his answer.

All these silences constituted the narrative fissures, the cracks in childhood psychic wholeness. Neither of these people really talked about this period of their lives. But there was always a feeling of something unsaid and secret in the family. There was another kind of silence. After the collapse of the USSR, when intensive international contacts began and we were invited to participate in discussions, the members of our delegations usually remained silent, which greatly surprised our partners. It was the fear of "coming forward," saying "wrong" as expected, and being punished – a learned colonial habit of not having a voice.

The Unconscious

With more than 300 years of Russian colonial influence on Ukraine, where three generations of Ukrainians were formed within the Soviet totalitarian trauma, and they have no other social experience to go by, all they know is trauma (Plokhy, 2023; Snyder, 2010). From generation to generation, we pass on this code of trauma, and it is deeply embedded in our unconscious. A kind of fixation on trauma can be found reflected in many Ukrainian traditions. Most of our traditional folk songs are sad. In art, Ukraine is depicted as raped, suffering, and one in need of liberation. The themes of defeat, death, violent death, and exile are present in arts and music. These themes are also found in works of Ukrainian poets, past and present. In recent history, after the events on the Maidan, the most popular Ukrainian song included central themes of dying in exile ("Plyve kacha"). The Suffering and Dying Hero has remained the main character and central archetype of our collective unconscious. This experience brings before the world a deep nature of transgenerational trauma, something which I grew up with.

My Unconscious

Stunningly, it is just in working on this contribution, I actually remembered my other identity outside of clinician and scholar – that of a poet. In my poetry, I also write about Ukraine, passive and tortured, captive, chained and crucified, waiting to be released. And I write about the earth, which knows no rest for hundreds of years and lays many sons in the graves, and I write about scars because trauma is a scar (Nalyvaiko, 2023).

Colonial Trauma

Ukraine bears many scars from small and large historical traumas, as noted above and shared in my story. The longest of them, lasting for centuries, is the colonial trauma caused by Russia. The term colonial trauma denotes both the political nature and collective impact of the trauma that Indigenous [local] communities endure (Mitchell, 2019).

Colonialism has been defined as "the takeover of territory, appropriation of material resources, exploitation of labor and interference with political and cultural structures of another territory or nation" (Mitchell, 2019, p. 2). Colonialism has also been defined by practices of cultural genocide, the spread of deadly diseases, the banning of Indigenous languages, forced assimilation and the illegalization of social, cultural, and spiritual practices (Paradies, 2016).

The manifestation of the colonial legacy was explored by Frantz Fanon, psychiatrist and political philosopher, who was born on the Caribbean island of Martinique, which was then a French colony (Gordon, 2015). Fanon has been described as "the most influential anticolonial thinker of his time" (Jansen & Osterhammel, 2017, p. 164). In his book *Black Skin, White Masks*, Fanon (1959/2016) sought to examine colonialism through psychoanalytical lenses. The colonial relations described by Fanon have a lot in common with the situation of Ukrainians in the Russian-Soviet context, where Ukrainians could "pass for a white man" if they renounced their identity and accepted the Russian-Soviet identity and ideology, articulates the Ukrainian scholar Mykola Riabchuk (2020), finding many parallels with the colonial experience analyzed by Fanon with the Ukrainian experience of Russian colonialism (Riabchuk, 2020).

Fanon analyzed the ways in which colonization captures the minds, bodies, and social institutions of the colonized nation. The situation investigated by Fanon is not unfamiliar to Ukrainians, suggested Riabchuk. It always starts the same way: with military force: with arms, weapons, economic subjugation, and additionally – with cultural subjugation. Ukrainians exemplify the behavior described by Fanon about the colonized subject: namely, in order to survive, they attempt to unconsciously identify themselves with the colonizer. With the years of colonization, natives not only get used to looking at themselves through the eyes of the colonizers but also uncritically assimilate their view, internalize it as "normal" – with all its Russian colonial stereotypes and suprematist prejudices. To a large extent, literature contributes to the formation of such a view.

This is emphasized by Eva Thompson in her book *Imperial knowledge: Russian literature and colonialism* (Thompson, 2000), where she presents a broad view of the cultural colonial expansion of Russia, analyzing Russian literature.

According to Mitchell (2019), "You don't come with guns anymore; you come with briefcases and we kill ourselves" (p. 257) in the voice of Raymond Quock, a Yukon Tlingit/Talhtan man. This haunting phrase reveals the perverse power of colonialism and the pervasive impact of internalized oppression. Researchers studying Native American and Canadian populations are likewise finding broad effects among children and grandchildren of survivors of massive cultural oppression. Thus, a group of scientists examined studies looking at the intergenerational effects of Indian residential schools, institutions run by the Canadian government from the 1880s until the mid-1990s. Eliminating the "Indian problem" was the aim of the schools, according to original government texts. The schools provided a substandard education and taught native children to be ashamed of their languages, cultural beliefs, and traditions (Bombay et al., 2014).

The local language and the signifiers of cultural affiliation associated with it suffer a particularly devastating effect. Stigmatization, humiliation, and marginalization of the national language become key elements of the subjugation of the natives, to the extent that in some families, the use of the local language is completely prohibited, and mothers scold their children for using it, describes Fanon (Fanon, 1959/2016). Language, like skin, is the most visible signifier of belonging to the indigenous nation and, therefore, becomes the object of symbolic and sometimes physical aggression. Accordingly, it is quite natural to want to get rid of this uncomfortable, dangerous element – to hide, keep silent, renounce, forget. Ukraine's national language has become a sort of stigma. It is the most obvious sign of belonging to the "worse" world, to the lower race of rural primitives, the lowest caste of collective farm slaves, marginalized in their impoverished villages, deprived even of their passports, represented backwardness (by analogy with Fanon's jungle).

"All prestigious, modern, fashionable, and bright had to be in Russian" (Riabchuk, 2020). In schools, children are used to being ridiculed for their "dialect." The nicknames used by the colonizers to describe the local population have a distinctly humiliating background: they evoke either animalistic associations or directly indicate mental or moral inferiority. As a result, the colonized, or the people subjected to colonization, in whose souls an inferiority complex has nested as a result of the death of their own cultural identity, come face to face with the language of the colonizer with the culture of the metropolis. The colonized can rise above the status of supposed savages, above their "jungles," only to the extent of assimilating metropolitan cultural standards (Fanon, 1959/2016).

The genocidal process of banning and destroying the Ukrainian language, which was called "linguicide," continued for centuries. Russian colonial policy systematically attempted to eliminate the Ukrainian language, which has survived over a hundred prohibitions and suppressions launched first by the Russian Empire and then by the Soviet Union. These prohibitions included the notorious Valuev Circular of 1863 (i.e., the decree issued by Piotr Valuyev, Minister of Internal Affairs of the Russian Empire), which banned the publication of all popular literature, including textbooks and religious texts in Ukrainian, officially denied the very existence of the Ukrainian language, stating explicitly "a separate Ukrainian language never existed, does not exist, and shall not exist" (Dibrova, 2017, p. 129). It was followed by the Ems Ukaz of 1876 (Dibrova, 2017), which extended the prohibition to imports of any Ukrainian books into the territory of the Russian Empire from abroad, the creation of original works in Ukrainian, making translations from foreign languages into Ukrainian, and even the printing of text into musical notes. The colonial policy of Ukraine's total Russification found its consistent and systematic continuation in the USSR. From 1622 to 2012, legislative acts were issued banning Ukrainian literature, Ukrainian theater, and Ukrainian translations, up to the complete denial of the existence of the Ukrainian language, decree on academic thesis defense only in Russian language and only in Moscow (1970), decree on privilege for the school teachers of Russian language (15% salary increase) – 1978, decree on Russian language classes increase in the school curriculum (1984) (Nalyvaiko, 2023).

Thus, since each language is a certain vision of the world and a certain way of thinking and is the identification code of every people, its renunciation and replacement by metropolitan one also causes worldview disorientation and an eclectic mentality. Fanon notes that this pushes the colonized peoples into a constant struggle with their own image, and prompts them to live in a split, which turns out to be extremely neurotic (Fanon, 1959/2016).

Personal Experience

When I was a child preparing for school, my parents were forced to send me to a Russian-speaking school in order to study a "normal" language, not a "peasant's" one. In order to survive, one of the coping strategies was full acceptance of the "rules of the game" of the system, phenomenologically experienced as the desire "to be like others." For more than 15 years, I was the only Ukrainian-speaking lecturer at one institute of psychoanalysis in Kyiv. In the whole of Ukraine, there were just a few of Freud's texts translated into Ukrainian; almost all of them were in Russian. Since the beginning of the large-scale invasion, precisely because of the unwillingness to identify with the invader through language, the majority of Ukrainians very quickly returned to their native Ukrainian language. In addition to language, a subcolonial nation is deprived of its history, culture, continuity of development, national myth, and national heroes. Fanon emphasizes that it has no valuable culture, no civilization, no long historical past (Fanon, 1959/2016).

To have a historical past means to have roots, sustainability, and continuity; it means to have a father who carries the idea of the primary stage and creation. Exploring Algeria's colonial legacy, Lazali's (2021) Colonial Trauma "offers a new myth of the primal scene of colonization, where there is not a murder of the father by his jealous sons but the disappearance of the father by the colonial invader" (in Chamberlin, 2023, https://www.journal-psychoanalysis.eu/articles/book-review-essay-colonial-trauma-a-study-of-the-psychic-and-political-consequences-of-colonial-oppression-in-algeria-by-karima-lazuli/).

A disappearance is not a murder – the Algerian "father" was not recognized by his vanquisher (Lazali suggested that the belief that North Africa has no history or culture is the "founding myth of colonialism," which the violence it justifies makes real), and he is consequently incapable of being either commemorated or forgotten" (in Chamberlin, 2023, https://www.journal-psychoanalysis.eu/articles/book-review-essay-colonial-trauma-a-study-of-the-psychic-and-political-consequences-of-colonial-oppression-in-algeria-by-karima-lazuli/). This colonial law of murder tries to "wipe out the culture to such an extent that this legacy can only appear as a blank space – a blank space expressed through a lack and excess to memory" (Lazali, 2021, p. 72). Such "a… "blank space" …forms the pathogenic nucleus that depersonalizes the [...] subject" (p. 72). It is the non-space of an extermination, a tabula rasa, a violence without traces and without tombs (Chamberlin, 2023).

It is the Russia's extermination toward Ukraine. "The complete liquidation of the Ukrainian state and its absorption by the Russian Federation" (Medvedev, 2024a) recently announced by Russian authorities, meaning the end of Ukraine as a sovereign and independent state in any borders. Russian psychoanalysis also makes a significant contribution to the formation of such a Russian colonial discourse. Yakushko (2023) who reviewed contributions by Russian psychoanalysts in service to Kremlin aggression, stated that "among the leading Russian psychoanalysts, similar to the period of Nazism, there are open propagandists of Russian military aggression and its justification"(p. 17). In their publications, quite shocking stories are presented, where Ukrainians are depicted as victims of their underdeveloped political and cultural environment, which has turned them to permanent fascism (i.e., the eternal "Nazism") (Yakushko, 2023), and the opinion is also expressed that one of the few "solutions" that Russia has in relation to Ukraine is to "continue to try to force one nation to live according to another nation's worldview" (Yakushko, 2023, p. 17).

These occurrences remain in line with the present-day Russian entitlement ideology to maintain "Russkiy Mir" ("Russian World" – the term actively pushed globally by Russian propaganda). It assumes that the so-called Russian "world" is the social totality associated with language, traditions, and history. According to its adherents, Russia has a unique mission to protect "Russkiy Mir" across the world. Their aim is to promote the Russian language and culture worldwide and form the Russian World as a global project (Kudors, 2010). The idea is that "those who *speak* Russian in their everyday life—also *think* Russian, and as a result—*act* Russian" (Kudors, 2010, p. 2). Since belonging to a cultural-linguistic group is considered to be the main determinant of one's belonging to the "Russian World," its boundaries are not strictly delimited. This characteristic in turn allows Russian federal authorities to target their policy of "protecting compatriots' interests at a broad group of foreign countries' citizens" (Kudors, 2010, p. 3).

Lazali (2021) in *Colonial Trauma*, proposed to examine the colonial legacy from the point of view of the "LRP bloc" (i.e., a fusion of language, religion, and politics) (p. 245). The meaning the erosion of the native language, along with religion and politics, mixing it with the language of the colonizer, religion, and politics of the colonizer are designed to lead to dissolution. Given the Ukrainian context of Russia appropriating Ukrainian history and culture, the "LHC" block can be considered, where H means history, C means culture.

> We could add a variation of Lazali's "LRP bloc" concept and propose the existence of an "RSI bloc," a fusion (instead of knotting) of the real, symbolic, and imaginary that supersedes any neurotic, perverted, or psychotic construction of existence—instead, the subject of colonial violence lives on the constant verge of dissolution.
>
> (Chamberlin, 2023, https://www.journal-psychoanalysis.eu/articles/book-review-essay-colonial-trauma-a-study-of-the-psychic-and-political-consequences-of-colonial-oppression-in-algeria-by-karima-lazuli/)

The denial or appropriation of historical heritage has been going on for centuries. The pieces of Ukrainian history from ancient times, when Ukraine was, and there was no Russia yet, are appropriated by Russia in order to artificially create their heritage. For instance, the Ukrainian Princess Anna, who later became the French queen, has been included in Russian textbooks on history as a "Russian queen," as well as Volodymyr the Great – Prince of Kyiv and ruler of Kyivan Rus, famous Ukrainian artists Kazymyr Malevych and Illya Repin, and a lead rocket engineer in the USSR, Sergiy Korolev – to mention just a few names expropriated by Russian colonialism. In fact, the history of Ukraine was almost excluded from the pupils' and university curriculum in Soviet schools.

Trauma of Holodomor

The long stay of Ukrainians under the influence of colonial trauma, in my opinion, enabled and aggravated the course of subsequent collective traumas, which were caused/created by totalitarianism. The cruelest of them, termed "one of the most traumatic events in the history of Ukraine" (Gorbunova & Klymchuk, 2020, p. 35) was the mass artificial starvation known as Holodomor (from Holod – "starvation," mor – "death").

Personal Experience

Since childhood, I absorbed the inevitable family truth that bread is holy. You can never throw it away, and you always must finish your meal, even if you are full. This belief is a national indisputable truth that is being passed from generation to generation among Ukrainians. This statement sounds like beautiful wisdom. However, the origins of this wisdom are unfortunately sad. This teaching stems from a collective fear of starvation caused by the Holodomor genocide in Soviet Ukraine in 1932–33, which still affects Ukrainians around the world. You always have to have something "in storage."

The Holodomor, recognized by many as a genocide, serves as a particularly potent source of collective pain. It was the largest man-made famine in Ukraine's history (the number of victims reached 4–7 million, according to different calculations). Much historical evidence indicates that the Holodomor was purposely organized to accomplish the Ukrainian genocide (Bilinsky, 1999). The intentional nature of the famine, coupled with the Soviet government's denial of the tragedy and the suppression of information, has contributed to a deep sense of injustice and grief that persists to this day. This event is not merely a historical fact but a wound that continues to affect the descendants of survivors, shaping their perceptions of trust, security, and national identity.

In the mid-to-late 2000s, Western scholar (Bezo & Maggi, 2015) lived and worked in Ukraine when Bezo began noticing a kind of social hostility and mistrust among the population. It was subtle, which is difficult to grasp for someone who has not been here for a long time. In his conversations with people, Bezo heard references to the Holodomor, the mass starvation of millions of Soviet Ukrainians from 1932 to 1933, considered by many to be an intentional genocide orchestrated by Joseph Stalin's regime. Wondering if and how this horrific event continued to resonate with the people, Bezo conducted a qualitative pilot study of 45 people from three generations of 15 Ukrainian families: those who had lived through the Holodomor, their children, and their grandchildren. People spontaneously shared what they saw as transgenerational impacts from that time, including risky health behaviors, anxiety and shame, food hoarding, overeating, authoritarian parenting styles, high emotional neediness on the part of parents, and low community trust and cohesiveness – what many described as living in "survival mode" (Bezo & Maggi, 2015, p. 87). Bezo noted that it seemed as if each generation, passing on experience to another, gave instructions not to trust others, and not to trust the world.

The events of 1932–1933, the silence that existed in society on the discussion of this topic, blocked the emotions of the survivors for a long time. Such powerful injuries do not heal with time, but leave their mark on the psyche, have an impact on behavior and lifestyle. The most common family behavioral strategies of descendants of Holodomor victims showed proper feeding, substantial food storage, and regular health check-ins. The most common respondent attitudes comprised a distrust of authority, disappointment with the government, and a priority of family needs over community needs (Gorbunova & Klymchuk, 2020).

The founder of the *International Center for the Study, Prevention and Treatment of Multigenerational Legacies of Trauma* Yael Danieli stated that massive traumas like these affect people and societies in multidimensional ways (Danieli, 1988). There are five factors of the Holodomor described by Masliuk (2010) that provoked psychological changes that could have been inherited: information deprivation (i.e., people did not know the extent of the starvation and the real aims of the Soviet government), confinement (i.e., people did not have the flexibility to escape from their regions), famine (i.e., there was insufficient food for survival), a ban on spiritual practices (i.e., people were required under threat of death to maintain only communist ideology), and the destruction of traditions (e.g., the tradition of mutual help and support) (Gorbunova & Klymchuk, 2020). However, whatever devastating consequences of the Holodomor could be, we cannot say that all worldview attitudes and behavioral strategies were caused only by the Holodomor. The whole totalitarian colonial system and concomitant propaganda distorted the moral and psychological health of Ukrainians, who have suffered a number of traumatic events in their history.

Volkan and Javakhishvili (2022) theorized that in societies that are treated inhumanely due to political systems, such as totalitarian regimes in former communist countries, even when political and legal systems change, and traumatizing elements within the society are removed, individual and societal responses to the previously existing and devastating political system do not disappear overnight. Depending on the severity of the traumatizing events and how long they lasted, the influence of the shared trauma on the victimized group and their descendants may continue for decades. The current ongoing war is another massive collective trauma of the Ukrainian nation. But, although cruel and bloody, this war demonstrated the ability of Ukrainians to overcome trauma. At the 53rd IPA Congress in Cartagena, Colombia, in a speech entitled *Mind in the Line of Fire*, Alderdice pondered:

> On February 24, 2022, the world witnessed the beginning of another historically significant conflict – Russia's invasion of Ukraine. The outcome remains uncertain, but despite Russia's military, economic, and

> numerical superiority, Ukrainians have demonstrated remarkable resistance. How do we explain why great powers with ever more sophisticated and deadly weapons —— are no longer winning wars?
>
> (online)

Alderdice related these processes to the "will to fight" (Alderdice, 2024, https://lordalderdice.com/index.php/2024/08/07/defence-not-war-must-be-the-priority/).

In reading this quote I consider the Hero archetype – a Hero who fights and dies and who is at the core of the Ukrainian unconscious. However, as all archetypes are ambivalent, the archetype of the Hero contains not only sacrifice, but also the idea of victory. Thus, this "will to fight," the sense behind it, together with social cohesion and international support, is creating a new experience of coping with the trauma of the ongoing war. Moreover, because none of the five factors of Masliuk's (2010) qualification of inherited trauma are characteristic of this war: information deprivation (people have access to all kinds of information), confinement (people have the flexibility to escape from their regions), famine (there is plenty of food), a ban on spiritual practices (people are able to follow any kind of practice), and the destruction of traditions (the traditions are followed) combined with the society acknowledgment, this war trauma, processed, mourned, and symbolized, will linger as a scar, and will not hurt, but will only be a mark of memory for the next generations.

References

Abrams, M. S. (1999). Intergenerational transmission of trauma: Recent contributions from the literature of family systems approaches to treatment. *American Journal of Psychotherapy*, 53(2), 225–231.

Alderdice, J. (2023). Mind in the Line of Fire. 53rd Congress of the International Psychoanalytical Association on 26th July 2023 in Cartagena, Colombia. https://lordalderdice.com/index.php/2024/08/07/defence-not-war-must-be-the-priority/

Bar-On, D., Eland, J., Kleber, R. J., Krell, R., Moore, Y., Sagi, A., … & Van Ijzendoorn, M. H. (1998). Multigenerational perspectives on coping with the holocaust experience: An attachment perspective for understanding the developmental sequelae of trauma across generations. *International Journal of Behavioral Development*, 22(2), 315–338.

Bezo, B., & Maggi, S. (2015). Living in "survival mode:" Intergenerational transmission of trauma from the Holodomor genocide of 1932–1933 in Ukraine. *Social Science & Medicine*, 134, 87–94.

Bilinsky, Y. (1999). Was the Ukrainian famine of 1932–1933 genocide? *Journal of Genocide Research*, 1(2), 147–156.

Brave Heart, M. Y. H., & Chase, J. (2011). Historical trauma among indigenous peoples of the Americas: Concepts, research, and clinical considerations. Journal of Psychoactive Drugs, 43(4), 282–290.

Brave Heart M. Y., & DeBruyn, L. M. (1998). The American Indian holocaust: Healing historical unresolved grief. *American Indian and Alaska Native Mental Health Research*, 8(2), 56–78.

Chamberlin, C. (2023). Book review essay: "Colonial Trauma: A Study of the Psychic and Political Consequences of Colonial Oppression in Algeria" by Karima Lazuli. *European Journal of Psychoanalysis*, 10(1). https://www.journal-psychoanalysis.eu/articles/book-review-essay-colonial-trauma-a-study-of-the-psychic-and-political-consequences-of-colonial-oppression-in-algeria-by-karima-lazuli/.

Cherepanov, E. (2020). *Understanding the transgenerational legacy of totalitarian regimes: Paradoxes of cultural learning*. Routledge.

Danieli, Y. (1988). *International Handbook of Multigenerational Legacies of Trauma*.

Dibrova, V. (2017). The Valuev Circular and the end of Little Russian literature. *Kyiv-Mohyla Humanities Journal*, (4), 123–138.

Evans-Campbell, T. (2008). Historical trauma in American Indian/Native Alaska communities: A multilevel framework for exploring impacts on individuals, families, and communities. *Journal of Interpersonal Violence*, 23(3), 316–338.

Fanon, F. (1959/2016). Black skin, white masks. In W. Longhofer, and D. Winchester (Eds.), *Social theory re-wired. New Connections to Classical and Contemporary Perspectives* (pp. 394–401). Routledge.

Gorbunova, V., & Klymchuk, V. (2020). The psychological consequences of the Holodomor in Ukraine. *East/West: Journal of Ukrainian Studies*, 7(2), 33–68.

Gordon, L. R. (2015). *What Fanon said: A philosophical introduction to his life and thought*. Fordham University Press.

Grand, S., & Salberg, J. (Eds.). (2016). *Trans-generational trauma and the other: Dialogues across history and difference*. Taylor & Francis.

Halbwachs, M. (2020). *On collective memory*. University of Chicago Press.

Jansen, J. C., & Osterhammel, J. (2017). *Decolonization: A short history*. Princeton University Press.

Kudors, A. (2010). Russian World'—Russia's Soft Power Approach to Compatriots Policy. *Russian Analytical Digest*, 81(10), 2–4.

Lazali, K. (2021). *Colonial trauma: A study of the psychic and political consequences of colonial oppression in Algeria*. John Wiley & Sons.

Masliuk, A. M. (2010). Riznovydy depryvuiuchykh chynnykiv podii holodomoriv v Ukraini pershoi polovyny XX stolittia [Varieties of depriving factors of the events of the Holodomor in Ukraine in the first half of the XX century]. *Scientific notes of the GS Kostyuk Institute of Psychology of the Academy of Pedagogical Sciences of Ukraine*, 38, 238–246.

Medvedev, D. (2024a). https://censor.net/ua/n3478672

Medvedev, D. (2024b). https://nv.ua/ukr/world/geopolitics/medvedyev-viklav-sim-punktiv-pro-kapitulyaciyu-ukrajini-i-formulu-miru-rf-analiz-novini-rosiji-50401332.html.

Mitchell, T. (2019). Colonial trauma: Complex, continuous, collective, cumulative and compounding effects on the health of Indigenous peoples in Canada and beyond. *International Journal of Indigenous Health*, 14(2), 74–94.

Nalyvaiko, N. (2023). Language metamorphoses as representations of subjectivity. Ukraine. Dairy of war. *Ukrainian Psychoanalytic Journal*, 1(1), 27–31. https://doi.org/10.32782/upj/2023-1-5

Plokhy, S. (2023). *The Russo-Ukrainian war: The return of history*. WW Norton & Company.

Riabchuk, M. (2020). https://www.radiosvoboda.org/a/mizhnarodna-konferentsija-ukrajinistiv/30972753.html

Salberg, J. (2017). The texture of traumatic attachment. In J. Salberg and S. Grand (Eds) *Wounds of history: Repair and resilience in the trans-generational transmission of trauma* (pp. 77–99). Routledge

Thompson, E. M. (2000). Imperial knowledge: Russian literature and colonialism. Westport, CT, and London: Greenwood.

Volkan, V., & Javakhishvili, J. D. (2022). Invasion of Ukraine: Observations on leader-followers relationships. *The American Journal of Psychoanalysis*, 82(2), 189–209.

Yakushko, O. (2023). Psychoanalysis and war: Histories of theorizing, resistance and support for war violence. *Ukrainian Psychoanalytic Journal*, 1(1), 14–20. https://doi.org/10.32782/upj/2023-1-3

Chapter 2

Phenomenology of Psychic Processes and Relationships in Wartime Ukraine

Valeriy Dorozhkin

Russia's full-scale invasion of Ukraine affected all the elements and processes that shape society. In particular, new powerful movements and associations have appeared, including various volunteer organizations and territorial defense of communities. Ordinary families felt a significant impact, and they began the process of rebuilding relationships, there were changes in the processes of growing up of children, some of whom grew up instantly, others, on the contrary, reacted by regressing. Residents of Ukraine have re-evaluated everyday things (e.g., as the cohabitation of unfamiliar people within the same house, understanding of comfort), and changed values (e.g., from individualization to grouping; from the accumulation of resources to the value of help). The collective subject of society itself has changed. During the first one and a half years of the war, the society was like a monolith, and only in the last six months the difference in views and differentiation of different layers of the population became noticeable. The invasion had a significant impact on relations in society. For example, most of the glass ceilings had disappeared. This became especially noticeable in the first year of the war when almost any resident could get to the head of his community and influence management decisions. In general, public hearings have gained considerable importance, and the government has turned to society with a human face and listens to and takes public opinion into account.

A certain percentage of the population also discussed the ethical possibility of buying expensive things (i.e., apartments, cars) during the war. The public felt such a strong collective guilt that they considered it inadmissible to spend money on anything other than donations and assistance to the Armed Forces of Ukraine. Questions of ordinary pleasures, such as entertainment, recreation, gym classes, and celebrating public and personal

DOI: 10.4324/9781032660257-3

holidays, became debatable. Even the Christmas tree has caused such strong public resistance that in most Ukrainian cities it has been refused for the second year in a row.

The war also caused changes in the psycho-emotional states of the collective subject. It went through such phases, as anxiety-affective (before the start of the invasion), panic (the first weeks of the invasion), paranoid-schizoid (from June 2022 to June 2023), and depressive (from the fall of 2023 to now). The change in psycho-emotional states shows that society learned to live during the war and is growing psychologically (Pustovoyt, 2023). However, this very change points to certain complexities and internal problems facing the public. In particular, from anxiety and emotional reactions, the population moved to split into "own-other". Now, on the contrary, society is experiencing a complex range of feelings, which is associated with the most visible figures and social institutions. Thus, distrust and dissatisfaction in the population increased, and a large number of social divisions arose according to various criteria and signs (i.e., military-non-military; there are dead relatives or not; there are among relatives those who were or are in captivity or not; one of the relatives participates in volunteer movements or not).

Some people felt such a compelling call from a society that they radically changed their lives. Some of them joined the territory defense or the armed forces, and others engaged in volunteer work collecting and sorting stuff and began weaving camouflage nets and dismantling rubble from rocket attacks. Since the beginning of the war, volunteer movements in gray areas have intensified (e.g., volunteers provide necessary things and medicine to people, animal volunteers help animals on the frontline territory). In general, gray areas have become a symptom of war. They indicate violated borders and, as a result, lawlessness, lack of authority, or clear rules in these territories.

Interestingly, breaking through borders led to an increase in their number. Currently, in Ukraine there are geographical borders of the country and frontiers, which separate the territory under control from the occupied, time limits have appeared (i.e., the curfew), political and positional borders between patriots and collaborators, air borders where civilian planes cannot fly, but where the rockets come from. The expansion of borders and frontiers is also associated with various types of invasions. They are caused by traitors, saboteurs, and informational psychological operations. Society needs to isolate it and keep it safe. By the third year of the war, people had learned to live in peculiar cocoons-containers, where only their circle was allowed. For some, it is broad and covers the whole society, for others it is narrowed to individual families or only themselves.

Relationships in therapy have also transformed. This became possible due to certain changes that affected the ethics of society. First, the law prohibiting cooperation with citizens and companies of Russia was adopted (as of June 24, 2022), after which therapists who until that moment were still working online with Russian clients or were supervised by Russian colleagues broke off relations. Secondly, the new ethics required transparency of positions and grouping. It also affected psychoanalysts. After many discussions in various therapeutic associations, the analysts decided that, first of all, they are citizens of their country. Therefore, they began to express their opinion, write about their feelings, provide more information about themselves in social networks, and, in general, took a more supportive and humane position toward analysands. Of course, this is a violation of the classic mirror position, but these changes created a safe space amid the chaos of war and provided the conditions for further self-disclosure of analysands (Dorozhkin, 2023a; Lagutin, 2023).

The therapeutic practice allowed those involved in it not only to withstand all the hardships and troubles of wartime but also became a tool for collecting and analyzing information. In the two years since the beginning of Russia's invasion of Ukraine, psychoanalysts have studied the psychological situation in society through private practice, support groups, supervision groups, participation in intervention groups and conferences, speeches at meetings of representatives of donor and public organizations. Along with the listed forms of work, I directly received and analyzed information as a manager and one of the psychotherapists within the framework of the Psychologists at War project, which lasted from August 2022 to September 2023. For more than a year, project specialists worked in the de-occupied territories and places close to the front line. Psychological work was carried out with people affected by the occupation, displaced persons, volunteers, community leaders, and local self-government bodies. A total of 29 specialists participated in the project, including representatives of the psychoanalytic approach, art therapists working with adults and children, specialists in the methods of "positive psychotherapy", "cognitive-behavioral therapy", "psychodrama", "clay therapy", Gestalt therapy, family doctors, rehabilitation specialists, etc. During the period of work, our team provided 7532 individual consultations and conducted 97 groups for adults and children for 1164 people. We managed to visit 48 settlements in the de-occupied territories or near the front line and train a network of local psychologists there, who received from us the experience of providing crisis first aid and the ability to conduct group sessions of psychological support.

During the active phase of the project, we met in intervision groups, analyzed and discussed the results of observations, and studied the mental states that our specialists had to deal with. We wrote reports, summarized the results, and this made it possible to highlight some psychological phenomena that are characteristic of people who suffered from the war and its consequences.

The specificity of these phenomena and experiences lies in the fact that all of them have excessive intensity and brightness, are subjectively perceived as those that cover the psyche entirely, and to a certain extent compel action. In addition, the emotional component of these mental states prevails over the cognitive one, and from the outside, it is perceived as a kind of regression of the psyche. Another feature that I have researched since mid-April 2022 is that most of the people who needed psychological support were in such a mental state that they did not have the internal ability and resources to seek help (Dorozhkin, 2023b). Such people also refused to work online or by phone. First of all, we are talking about vulnerable categories of the population who were in temporarily occupied territories and were subjected to violence, pressure, torture, rape, humiliation, etc. It was also found that the victims experienced such strong emotions of confusion, despair, helplessness, loss of self-esteem, difficulties with self-identification, high levels of anxiety, and depressive states that these experiences prevented any social contact. Even after the liberation of the occupied territories, such people did not have the mental resources to independently turn to crisis services or individual psychotherapists; they experienced difficulties with establishing and restoring contacts, and, in fact, needed re-socialization. That is why mobile teams of our specialists came to the affected communities and worked directly on the ground. There I collected and then described most of the phenomena that will be presented below.

Phenomena Related to the Change in the Ratio of Peaceful and Military Life

It is worth saying that the invasion of Ukraine did not begin on February 24, 2022, but with the annexation of Crimea, which took place on February 27, 2014, when the central authority, the Verkhovna Rada of Crimea, was seized. At that time, I lived in the Crimea (where I was born and grew up), in the administrative center of this region – the city of Simferopol. The occupation of Crimea forced me to leave my job at the university, leave my private practice, friends, and relatives, and move to Kyiv. This was my way of expressing my disagreement with the fact that Russia began to do in Crimea. By the way, out of 22 members of the Faculty of Psychology of Tavriya University (Simferopol) after the annexation of Crimea, 6 teachers moved to different cities of Ukraine – 27% of the staff. Approximately the same picture took place in other departments and faculties. At that time, it was quite a radical step. At that time, they had not yet started killing and torturing dissenters, and there were no more than two dozen missing Crimeans. The occupation was relatively mild, compared to the modern war, and it gave rise to a significant wave of dissent in Crimea, protest actions, and huge queues at the only service where you can cancel your Russian citizenship, which was compulsorily assigned to everyone. All this happened even before the beginning of the active phase of annexation, namely until April 12, 2014, when Ukrainian patriots began to be killed masse in the east of the country.

I bring this small excursion into history to show that military operations came to Ukraine much earlier than the full-scale invasion, and by February 24, 2022, the population had already received a "vaccination against war" and learned to live in conditions of permanent hostilities. But until a full-fledged war began, for most people these actions took place "somewhere far in the east" and did not affect them directly. On the day of the invasion, almost all civilians felt a strong shock and it dramatically changed the ratio of peaceful and military life.

The War Became a Figure, and Everyday Life Went into the Background

The beginning of the war divided life into "before and after". And this is not just a phrase. Plans, style, and fulfillment of life have changed, relations with relatives from Russia have been canceled: here we are not even talking about distant relatives, but about parents, children, brothers, and sisters, property has been lost, loved ones have died. Undoubtedly, these experiences affected the psyche and experiences of people. People felt guilty for not being able to protect their loved ones and the country, for a certain time citizens forbade themselves joy, entertainment, and rest; everyday life faded into the background in thoughts and conversations, and war and related events took its place. All this led to the fact that a significant number of Ukrainians lost interest in everyday life. In therapy sessions, especially during the first year of the war, I repeatedly heard things like, “How can I talk about my own life when the war is going on and people are dying? My problems are not so important and have lost relevance”, “I am ashamed to complain when others die or lose everything”.

Another, but related to the previous, reaction manifested itself in the fact that some Ukrainians overestimated the peaceful world, values, and the usual order of things. People were confronted with the fragility of ordinary life. The revaluation of the world has gone in the direction of valuing momentary pleasures and the “here-and-now” moment, but it is also connected with the devaluation of the future, “which may not come”. Momentary pleasures became an attempt to overcome the realities of war and do not contradict the self-rejection of joy. On the contrary, they only emphasize the ambivalence of the psyche. Some citizens refused to enjoy; others heightened its fleeting presence in the moment. However, it is fundamental that all these joys essentially contain tragedy within them. They are not aimed at the future but are experienced as the enjoyment of the last day.

In my psychoanalytic practice, I noticed that the war continues not only outside, but also inside each analysand. It segments the self, splits it into parts, forms an internal battlefield, and makes certain parts of the identity the object of attacks. Thus, the war reinforces the internal division of the self. Two years after the beginning of the full-scale invasion, the described phenomena are manifested to a lesser extent than in the first months of the war, but some of them do not lose their intensity even now.

Everyday Presence of Objects that Traditionally Have Negative Semantics

Death

During the war, the average Ukrainian is constantly faced with the death of people they know and do not know. This happens in the news feeds of various social networks and conversations with friends. Death is present in the background and is set by the very fact of war, the arrival of missiles and drones, shelling. Civilians have learned to live every day as if it were their last, and appreciate every moment, which strengthens attention to a specific moment and themselves in it. The permanent presence of death intensifies emotions and makes them bright and unusual. At present, any feelings are tinged with death, so they are perceived as complicated, and sometimes as such, which cannot be gotten rid of due to their excess. Buchinska, one of the specialists of the project "Psychologists at War", articulated: "The fear of death ceased to be felt as something great and magical, but at the same time it did not become less significant. This created a sense of the presence of death in every day of life. And such a presence gives fullness and meaning" (Personal communication, 2022).

Death became a prominent figure in the everyday and this led to the fact that it seemed to challenge life, and … life also became a significant figure. At present, life is powerfully enhancing vitality and craving for everything related to it. By the way, such a view on the interaction of life and death is inherent in most of our people and supports analysands in psychotherapy.

Enemies

The presence of the enemy "there, on the front line" is supported by the feeling of their presence "here, deep in the rear". Such a phenomenon is not widespread among the military but is inherent in civilians. Ordinary people are busy looking for internal enemies because they cannot reach the external enemy, and they blame the one who is nearby. We are talking about displaced aggression, described for the first time by K. Lorenz (1967). I came across this phenomenon in Borodyanka, a small town in the north of the Kyiv region, which has undergone significant destruction. At the psychological support group, the residents of the city argued against the local and state authorities, deputies and officials, volunteers, and themselves. It seemed that they were hostile to the whole world. In groups elsewhere, I have repeatedly heard women conflict with their husbands for taking the wrong road and getting stuck/under fire at the start of the invasion; husbands resented their wives for taking a long time to pack, or for not going to the west of the country before the war began (i.e., when the husbands offered it to them); adult children were dissatisfied with their elderly parents and the fact that they, in general, did not want to go anywhere; parents were indignant at the children that the latter were involved in volunteer help at the risk of their lives. In many psychological support groups, participants blamed each other, and looked for enemies and traitors, but, at the same time, continued to be in contact with each other. This contact, in my opinion, is an important platform for restoring trust.

Among other things, I noticed that people preferred to appoint to the position of internal enemies those people to whom claims could be made and with whom dialogue was possible. That is why the occupiers were hardly talked about in the groups. They were tacitly perceived as real enemies. The hatred, anger, and contempt for them were so strong, that there were no words to express the feelings, so silence spoke more eloquently. However, the silence was a symptom, reflecting excess energy that shifted to loved ones. Observations showed that sometimes the search for culprits and traitors in the middle of individual families led to the fact that families could not withstand conflicts and fell apart.

Distrust

The imaginary and sometimes real presence of enemies nearby affects the emergence of another feeling – distrust. Distrust opposes the sense of unity and becomes another symptom of the ambivalent experiences during the war. It also contributed to the disillusionment of some people in the figures of those whom they attributed to the Great Others. Traditional objects of support could not protect a peaceful world, so their internal representatives experienced inflation, and people themselves began to look for new support (Velykodna, 2023). My experience, as well as the practice of psychotherapists who were involved in the work of the Psychologists at War project, showed that the public repeatedly changed its attitude toward symbolic parental figures: community leaders, the government, the president, God. Disappointment, resentment, anger, pride, respect, and suspicion replaced each other. The only Big Other, the attitude toward which almost did not fluctuate during the war, is the Armed Forces of Ukraine. The saying "I believe in the Armed Forces of Ukraine" even spread in society. In a certain sense, the Armed Forces of Ukraine have taken the place of God and for a year now have more than 90% of unchanged trust (according to the Sociological Group "Rating", 2023).

The revaluation and inflation of the figures of the Great Others has led to the fact that in many families there has been a revision of parental and male figures as protective. Unfortunately, it turned out that the protective function does not depend on whether a person is in the army or remains a civilian. If the sense of basic security is destroyed, there will always be room for suspicion. I am familiar with cases where women who went abroad accuse their military husbands of the fact that the latter abandoned them to their own devices and are not with them. On the contrary, there are stories where women are ashamed of their husbands if they do not go to defend the country. Both variants are not so widespread as to speak of trends, but they occur and have an impact on family relationships and dissatisfaction with each other. In extreme cases, such dissatisfaction leads to divorces.

Revaluation of the figures of the Great Others is connected not only with mistrust but also with a revision of values and priorities. What was significant to individuals became insignificant and vice versa. In many families, the process of revaluation proceeds unevenly and at different speeds, which increases the difference between worldviews and creates additional areas of conflict. The latter prompts partners to look for people closer in values and affects relationship satisfaction.

Spooky

The war and the events connected with it influenced the fact that the spooky was combined with pleasure. At the same time, it frantically came out of the unconscious, invaded the ego, and threatens to poison the ego, to change it with all the invasions of the spooky non-ego (Prokhasko, 2021). Contemplation of enemy corpses, torn bodies, and severed limbs, which are available to us in open Telegram channels, excess experiences of rage, fear, desire to kill, thirst for revenge, joy from the fact that our soldiers destroy enemies – all this changes the self, reformats it into something different – unfamiliar and threatening in relation to today's self.

The spooky carnival of the war caused derealization and partial depersonalization. Unfortunately, we have adapted to such everyday life, where city dwellers do not sleep at night due to sirens and powerful explosions, and in the morning contemplate burnt high-rise buildings, in which living people were still sleeping at night; we are supposedly used to the bodies of murdered people, burned cars, destroyed schools and shopping centers. But we still cannot come to terms with the thought that the same terrible story may happen to us tomorrow. And it can really happen. Currently, no one is safe from missiles that reach any remote place in the country. And we cannot accept everything that is happening now as normal life. We seem to have fallen into some terrible world brought about by the war and the occupying country: people sleep in the subway because it is the only reliable bomb shelter; in the middle of a frosty winter, cities remain without electricity, heating, and water – this is our reality during the war years. And this reality is not normal. It became like that thanks to repetition from day to day for two years now. But the most terrifying thing is not that people get used to the spooky, but that they learn to enjoy it. It is the pleasure of revenge, rage, and hatred. The pleasure of Thanatos and the energy of mortido. This is a true frenzy, where self meets all aspects of non-self that have invaded from within the unconscious. Undoubtedly, the new parts enriched the self, making it stronger – during the war, we need exactly this – but also changed the self, adding rigidity to it.

Caillois (1960) stated that during the war previously forbidden events become conventional, and the war itself is part of the sacred, has an archaic nature, and causes regression of the psyche of the subjects involved in it. The laws of wartime are different from the laws of peacetime. You can kill and enjoy killing enemies, you can be aggressive, you can swear, you can watch videos from the front marked with "special brutality". All these processes require other qualities of the soul – such features that are not used in peaceful times and are hidden in the archaic layers of the psyche.

Most of what happens during the war seems implausible and unreal to us – ordinary residents. However, with our own eyes or from street cameras, we saw and continue to see how the occupiers destroyed architectural monuments, killed children, young and old, men and women, raped and robbed. We are in contact with the spooky, and to endure it, we have to become frantic and tough. We split not only reality but also ourselves. Not only the military but also civilians take part in this sacred carnival. As the proverb says: everyone dances this tango of death. However, there is something that allows you to withstand all this load. I mean love and altruism.

Phenomena Related to the Peculiarities of Experiences during the War

Features of Emotions in Wartime, Love, and Altruism

Many Ukrainians in social networks and psychotherapy groups say that they have never felt such intensity of rage, hatred, anger, love, desire to help, compassion for others, and a sense of unity before. The level of emotions goes off the scale, it seems that they cover the entire psyche, and begin to dominate consciousness. A participant of one of the psychological support groups within the framework of the "Psychologists at War" project shared: "In peaceful life, people do not feel this way". From the outside, it looks like a kind of mental regression, when emotions rule over cognition, and the role of the observing and reflecting self is reduced. Such a state is inherent in childhood. Civilians are often unable to cope with their mental states and have only to witness the processes taking place in their psyche. At the same time, they have the feeling that there is no possibility to manage these processes. That is why people are full of emotions and become more impulsive.

Among the features of experiences during wartime, I include:

- unfolding of emotions against the background of war, which gives them additional
- energy and dynamics;
- confusion, mixing, and unification of emotions – this makes them more complex and
- composed of polar feelings, including hatred, rage, anger, despair, fear, sadness, sorrow,
- joy, admiration, respect, pride, and love;
- the high threshold for recognizing emotions.

The latter means that a significant part of the population experiences difficulties in revealing their own subtle emotions, and feelings become noticeable only when they gain a certain intensity. On the contrary, less pronounced emotions remain in the background perception, and to track and experience them, you need to do a lot of mental work. However, they affect and burden the mental states of people in wartime.

Such mental dynamics are additionally complicated by the fact that people feel self-identity, and continuity of themselves and do not notice changes. Blindness to the self performs a protective role, but it does not allow one to notice the growing gap, the gap between the present self, united with frenzy and various aspects of the non-self, and the past self. Nevertheless, there is one fundamental change that is visible to the naked eye – the emergence of new intense types of love.

Lacan (2017) theorized in one of his seminars that love is an unbearable truth about the lack of fundamental integrity of a split subject, which they seek to fill with the help of an object. During the war, not only the subject is split, but also the objects of love. In addition, a significant number of citizens have new love objects, including Ukrainianness, the Ukrainian nation, and the Motherland. Love for Ukraine is currently so strong that for its explanation it is appropriate to recall the ideas of the ancient Greeks about the forms of love, among which they distinguished: ludos, eros, mania, pragma, philia, philautia, storge, agape (Baird, 2010). Let me remind you that ludos, eros, mania, pragma, filia, and storge refer to different types of partner love; philautia is self-love, which, unlike narcissistic feelings and autoerotism, does not contain, in the understanding of the ancient Greeks, a negative connotation. On the contrary, agape is a feeling toward a collective or group subject, which is not directly sexualized, and, in modern language, is sublimation.

The results of the research we conducted as part of the "Psychologists at War" project showed that currently, most of the military and part of the civilians have experienced a change in their feelings of love. The role of the erotic component of this feeling decreased and gave way to friendly feelings, which grew and strengthened brotherly love (i.e., love for comrades in arms, who in the military hierarchy currently have a higher priority than one's husband or wife). Also, the supra-individual component of love, which is present in agape – a strong passion for Ukrainianness and the Motherland as a whole – has increased significantly. In our study, 20% of respondents feel agape feelings. These data coincide with two other observations. According to the first of them, each social group has 20% altruists (Ridley, 1995). Another corresponds to my assumption that 20% of people felt the forced call of society (Dorozhkin (Keiselman), 2016). It is this percentage that includes citizens who radically changed their lives and became soldiers or actively started volunteering, clearing rubble. The idea that agape replaced eros is also confirmed by surveys of military wives. A total of 80% of them note that the erotic component of the relationship with their husbands has been replaced by a friendly and valuable one.

Psychological Boundaries, Narcissistic Trauma, and War

War destroys boundaries. We are talking not only about the borders of the country but also about psychological boundaries and self-demarcation of the individual, using the concept of self-demarcation was proposed by Ammon (1984). The framework of ordinary life – everything that was permanent and usual – was also destroyed. People lost not only the usual meaning of life but also its form, changed it to forced resettlement and added ritualized actions to ordinary things: volunteering, daily scrolling through news on social networks, reactions to air alarms, when it is necessary to perform a certain set of permanent actions.

While working with psychological support groups, I encountered an amazing phenomenon. Along with the participants who experienced an unusual brightness of emotions, some live as if they have turned off their feelings. Such people comment on their condition as ego-dystonic, alien to them, caused by inner emptiness and burnout. The majority of such people are found among the categories of the population most affected by the war. They developed such a strong self-distinction between the cognitive and affective spheres that they almost stopped feeling emotions and protected themselves from feelings. This applies not only to the experiences that are caused by the traumatic events during the invasion and occupation but also to the emotions toward one's loved ones, partners, children, ordinary life, and oneself. Victims have a significantly increased threshold for recognizing what they are feeling at a particular moment in time. Their relations have become cold, functional, and dissociative. The most mentally traumatized people covered themselves with a crust of distrust. They feel alienated from others and avoid contact with them. Undoubtedly, this has a negative impact on the restoration of social ties in cities and villages that were under occupation and requires separate social and psychological work.

There is another phenomenon connected with boundaries. After the start of the war, some of the residents of Ukraine began to move the boundaries and self-demarcation (Nalyvaiko, 2023). Such internal processes affected the fluctuations of intimacy that a person is ready for, the change in the threshold of impulsivity of their reactions (i.e., from disinhibition to unnatural restraint), and the fluctuations in self-esteem and self-attitude. This category of people has become hardly recognizable to relatives, friends, acquaintances, and even to themselves.

All of the listed features point to the need to work out psychological boundaries and self-demarcations related to them, which, secondarily, restores the circulation of mental material not only between instances of the psyche but between people and the world. For many people from our country, such work gives them a chance to harmonize their personalities. In this sense, it is interesting that the invasion itself allowed Ukraine to start returning the territories to the borders of 2014. Although this happens due to the initial violation or destruction of the borders, it launched protective processes in society and individuals.

Another point related to the breaking of the boundaries concerns the blow into the narcissistic part of the personality of Ukrainians. This attack took place thanks to Russian propaganda, dehumanization of prisoners, and inhumane treatment of the population in the occupied territories of Kyiv, Sumy, Kharkiv, Chernihiv, and Kherson regions – all places where residents resisted. Among the questions that the citizens of our country asked at the beginning of the war were: "Why do the Russians have such a barbaric attitude toward us? Why do our relatives from the occupying country not believe us? Why are our architectural monuments, universities, schools, hospitals, kindergartens, shopping centers, and residential areas destroyed? How many civilians have to die so that the Western countries give us the necessary weapons and impose sanctions against the racist regime?"

Any answers to these rhetorical questions do not satisfy us, because they do not close the traumatic void in connection with the events. This is because the citizens of our country do not need information, but the healing of narcissistic trauma due to recognition, satisfaction, or victory. By the way, some questions fell away by themselves after our army liberated Kyiv, Sumy, Kharkiv, Chernihiv, and, partially, Kherson regions. But in relationships and self-attitude there is still a dystrophy of the healthy part of narcissism. We are shocked by the treacherous invasion of the Rashists and the narcissistic wound hurts. In the previous article, it was shown how important the narcissistic coloring of therapeutic support is at present (Dorozhkin, 2023a). It restores justice and humanity, which were destroyed by dehumanization in Russian propaganda and trampled by war (Yakushko, 2023).

Similar opinions are expressed by Rechkalova, a specialist in the project "Psychologists at war". She writes: "People are truly traumatized and bereft. If they are given a safe and empathetic space, they start talking about it. And people need recognition of their experience and normalization of feelings about it" (Personal communication, 2022). These processes indicate an immense need to restore the narcissistic part and rebuild a sense of self-respect (Velykodna, 2023). I would like to add that the situation has improved a little, a sense of dignity has been restored due to the significant number of victories of our army, and pride has arisen for our indomitable people and the country as a whole.

Phenomena Related to the Impact of War on the Growing up of Children

Children's upbringing was affected by the fact that the war posed the same questions to everyone, regardless of social status, gender, and age. These questions were focused on how to survive the invasion and how to protect the valuable. Many of the adults did not find the answers or found them later than their offspring. Therefore, the children had to find their understanding of the situation instead of their parents, according to the materials of support groups and individual consultations within the framework of the Psychologists at War project. I know of cases when minor children calmed down their parents during shelling, took them to a bomb shelter, found food and cooked food for the family, and even looked for safe ways to move around the country. Moreover, not adults, but children explained as they could what began to happen in the country after the start of the war.

I am far from thinking that such cases were numerous, but I know that they happened. Based on the materials of the groups, I managed to establish that the intensive growing up of children is connected with the presence/absence of regression in their parents. If adults defended themselves from the reality of war and regressed, then children took their place as parents. On the contrary, if parents, in their need to maintain control, took a too authoritarian and directive position in relation to children, then the latter regressed to the previous age. At the consultation of the specialists of the Psychologists at War project, parents came who said that their relatively big children (ages 10 to 15) had enuresis, attention disorders, children's fears (of darkness, being alone in a room), worries about loss of parents (e.g., a case when the child was afraid of losing eye contact with his mother), social phobia. These children did not have all the mentioned symptoms before the war.

Nechkina, a specialist in the project "Psychologists at War", systematizes the impact of the occupation and the consequences of the invasion on children in the following theses:

- currently, children do not have enough communication with their parents, even when it seems that it is enough;
- children are more sensitive to loud sounds (for example, thunder or the movement of chairs in other rooms);
- many parents in the de-occupied territories began to restrict their children from playing outdoors with other children due to the fear of losing the child;
- a large number of children in the de-occupied territories do not live their children's lives, but participate in following their parents and co-living adult life instead of their own. Nechkina calls the social phenomenon in which "children are alive, but not living" the syndrome of "viewing life through a protective glass" (Personal communication, 2022).

Intensive growing up of children requires changes in relations with parents. Currently, children need more partner relationships. They want recognition from their parents for the growing up that has happened to them. In modern Ukrainian families, this has become a challenge for both parents and children themselves.

Conclusions

Several important phenomena characterizing the mental state of individual and group subjects during the war are described. These phenomena are related to the fact that war destroys the built structure of the psyche and encourages the unconscious to rule. This happens due to feeding instincts and basic emotions. In turn, the dominance of the unconscious creates a special space into which the psyche of individual and collective subjects is placed. This space affects the attitude of people to each other, the peculiarities of communication and relationships in different social groups, and the specifics of inner experiences and mental phenomena. Family, group relationships, and self-relationships experienced a significant transformation. With the help of psychoanalytic methodology, it is possible to investigate these transformations and systematize them according to certain criteria.

References

Ammon, G. (1984). Die Bedeutung des Körpers im ganzheitlichen Verständnis der humanistischen Dynamischen Psychiatrie [The importance of the body under the holistic aspect of humanistic dynamic psychiatry]. *Dynamische Psychiatrie*, 17(4)[87], 339–356

Baird, F.E. (2010). *Philosophic classics: Ancient philosophy* (Vol. I). Routledge.

Caillois, R. (1960). *Man and the sacred*, trans. M. Barash. Free Press of Glencoe.

Dorozhkin, V. (2023a). Therapeutic relationships in wartime Ukraine. *Psychoanalytic Psychology*, 40(4). https://doi.org/10.1037/pap0000482

Dorozhkin, V. (2023b). Current war and its impact on the therapeutic relationship. *Ukrainian Psychoanalytic Journal*, 1(1). https://doi.org/10.32782/upj/2023-1

Dorozhkin (Keiselman), V. (2016). Hrani altruizma. [*Edges of altruism*]. Fenix. 320 p.

Lacan, J. (2017). *Formations of the unconscious: Book 5*: The seminar of Jacques Lacan. Polity Press.

Lagutin, V. (2023). Psychoanalysis "traumatized" by war. Four clinical illustrations of the vulnerability of the setting. *Ukrainian Psychoanalytic Journal*, 1(3). https://doi.org/10.32782/upj/2023-3-3

Lorenz, K. (1967). *On aggression*. Bantam Books.

Nalyvaiko, N. (2023). Borders and psychoanalysis in a time of war. *Psychoanalytic Psychology*, 40(4). https://doi.org/10.1037/pap0000485

Prokhasko, Y. (2021). Psykhoanaliz i suchasnist [*Psychoanalysis and modernity*]. Zbruč.

Pustovoyt, M. (2023). Interpreting crisis while in crisis (reflections on psychoanalytic work in hybrid warfare). *Ukrainian Psychoanalytic Journal*, 1(1). https://doi.org/10.32782/upj/2023-1-4

Ridley, M. (1995). *The red queen: Sex and the evolution of human nature*. Penguin Books.

Sociological Group "Rating." (2023). How the war changed me and the country. Summary of the year – 2023. Retrieved at https://www.ratinggroup.ua/en/news/kompleksne-dosl-dzhennya-yak-v-yna-zm-nila-mene-ta-kra-nu-p-dsumki-roku

Velykodna, M. (2023). A Psychoanalyst's experience of working in wartime: On choosing between bad options. *Psychoanalytic Psychology*, 40(4). https://doi.org/10.1037/pap0000480

Yakushko, O. (2023). Psychoanalysis and war: Histories of theorizing, resistance and support for war violence. *Ukrainian Psychoanalytic Journal*, 1(1). https://doi.org/10.32782/upj/2023-1

Chapter 3

Oedipal Conflicts During Wartime

War and the Infantile Fantasies

Yuliia Vizniuk and Elina Yevlanova

This chapter summarizes the experiences of the authors' joint work in the supervisory project "War Time Research" (Yevlanova, 2023), which was organized in response to the 2022 Russian invasion of Ukraine. At some point, it became apparent that with the change in the dynamics of military operations in Ukraine, the nature of complaints with which patients sought psychological help changed. If in the early months of the war, we mostly worked in the format of crisis counseling with our patients struggling to accept the new circumstances of life, then around 12 months later, patients started coming to psychoanalysts' offices, telling stories of the love dramas they experienced during that time. This allowed us to return to the format of psychoanalytic counseling. In the focus of this research, we decided to place the question of how and why war actualizes Oedipal conflicts, which until then could have been considered dormant in the emotional life of individuals under the pressure of repression.

We consider the concept of Oedipal conflict according to the views of Sigmund Freud and his followers (Freud, 1961; Freud & Strachey, 2001). Namely, every child has loving and hostile desires directed toward their parents. The regulation of erotic and aggressive impulses can take positive and negative forms. In the positive form, there is a desire for the death of the rival – the parent of the same sex, and sexual desire directed toward the parent of the opposite sex. In the negative form, there arises love for the parent of the same sex and jealousy and hatred toward the parent of the opposite sex.

The peak of these desires falls between the ages of 3 and 6 in the phallic phase of psychosexual development. In the latent period, they fade away, and in puberty, they become active again, culminating in a non-incestuous choice of object (Laplanche & Pontalis, 2018).

DOI: 10.4324/9781032660257-4

The Oedipal period marks a shift in the child's life from the logic of demand to the logic of desire, from dyadic mother-child relationships to triadic father-mother-child relationships. At its core lies the child's recognition of the nature of parental relationships and the fantasies dedicated to them. The realization that parents sleep together, not allowing the child to sleep nearby, can evoke the child's fantasy that the parents have left him to die. The desire to enter into rivalry with one of the parents for the right to possess the other becomes an inexhaustible source of fear of parental or one's death. Generally, it is during this period that the so-called terrifying children's nightmares appear, and children begin to ask questions about death. Fear of punishment for one's desires, the threat of castration, and the anxiety associated with it lay the groundwork for the formation of the castration complex, which develops differently in boys and girls (Lacan, 2011, Seminar 5). Exiting this period of life, the child receives identification with the parental object of the same sex.

Thus, the Oedipal complex is a structure that forms the basis of interpersonal relationships and the way the subject sees and appropriates a certain place in this structure. This is the basis for a child's entry into culture and is the foundation of neurotic psychopathology in its various manifestations (Freud & Strachey, 1986). Fantasies help the child experience difficult moments, reduce anxiety levels, find their answers to troubling questions, and restore injured narcissism. Primary infantile incestuous fantasies are repressed and replaced by "safe" fantasies. This is wonderfully illustrated by the story of Little Hans, about whom Freud (1955) suggested:

> In his attitude towards his father and mother Hans confirms in the most concrete and uncompromising manner what I have said in my Interpretation of Dreams and in my Three Essays with regard to the sexual relations of a child to his parents. Hans really was a little Oedipus who wanted to have his father "out of the way," to get rid of him, so that he might be alone with his beautiful mother and sleep with her.
>
> (p. 126)

Among the main stages of his recovery from a phobia, one can recall dreams about a plumber replacing a broken faucet and the fantasy of getting rid of the father by sending him on a trip to his mother, Hans's grandmother.

The function of childhood fantasizing, to which we owe the entire cultural heritage of humanity, never disappears. It manifests itself in adults in conscious and unconscious fantasies and always represents a sequence of scenes in which the subject is constantly present. Also, the main function of fantasizing is that any fantasy scene, like a dream, reflects desire, while prohibition is also present within it. This prohibition is ensured through primary psychological defenses: inversion, transformation into the opposite, projection, and denial.

In the realm of the Unconscious, there are no contradictions, denials, or time (Freud & Strachey, 1955). However, we experience a sense of time from the first months of life due to the presence or absence of the mother (Pavlovska, 2024). On October 4, 2023, at her speech at the Conference of the Division of Psychoanalytic Psychology and Psychotherapy of the National Psychological Association of Ukraine "Psychoanalysis on Time," psychoanalyst Nina Kokoilo made a presentation titled "The Tyranny of Time." According to her speech, a person experiences the past as "running time," the future as a hallucinatory dimension, and the present as an endless experience. The experience of time is always linked to the inevitability of death. This process caused the feeling of the tyranny of time, and frustration from the moment of birth. Perhaps, a person feels the tyranny of time most acutely in times of war; likewise, one can keenly feel during wartime how interconnected life and death are. The fear of death can lead a person to perceive life as an opportunity to do something new. If the urge for self-preservation, and erotic urges are actualized, the time split into "before and after" can be connected. Love is what can perform the function of linking time, providing life with new meanings related to the present and the future.

Below we include two examples from our clinical work that illustrate our observations on oedipal issues.

Clinical Examples

April 2023 (1 Year and 2 Months of the Full-Scale War)

"Better to do it today, as there's no certainty about tomorrow" – analysand's quote.

Mrs. O. is 34 years old, married with two preadolescent daughters, and owns her own business. We have known each other for a long time, or rather, this is her fourth attempt at therapy. The first time she came for a consultation was in 2019, seemingly to get acquainted and assess the therapist, but after some time, she requested couples therapy with her husband, and after its completion, she returned because she realized she had questions about herself that she wanted to address in individual therapy. Her request sounded like this: "I don't want to be like my mother." However, she interrupted the sessions, stating that she was moving to another city and didn't want to continue therapy online. When we decided to end our work, on the penultimate meeting, Mrs. O. confessed that she wanted to tell me something no one knew: that all these years she has been living with her husband, but she has been in love with another man.

Four years have passed. The war in Ukraine had been going on for over a year. Mrs. O. reached out with a desire to continue her therapy online. At the first session, she asked if the analyst remembered how she ended her previous therapy, stating that everything was fine then, but now everything had changed because the man she loved had reappeared in her life, and their relationship had resumed.

Family History of Mrs. O.

The families of Mrs. O. parents lived in nearby apartments. Her mother dated a man she loved deeply, but he betrayed her and married someone else. Afterward, the analysand's parents started a romantic relationship. Mrs. O.'s father came from a wealthy and influential family; his father held a high position in the city. Because of this, Mrs. O.'s mother's parents insisted they get married. Mrs. O. was born a year later.

When the analysand was 3 years old, her father went to study in another city, where he met a woman and started new relationships. The analysand's parents officially divorced when she was 4 years old. Her father remarried and had a daughter, and the analysand felt intense jealousy toward her. Her mother immediately began dating a man she loved before her father, who eventually divorced his wife and started living with them.

Mrs. O., her mother, and her stepfather lived in a small two-bedroom apartment with her maternal grandparents. The stepfather was a military doctor who came home on weekends. When he was absent, the analysand slept with her mother in one bed, and when he was present, she slept on a bed between her grandmother and grandfather. They lived like this until Mrs. O. entered university. Her memories of the family she grew up in were very sad: her mother always said they had little money, her grandmother suffered from diabetes and eventually went blind, and Mrs. O. partially cared for her. Her relationship with her stepfather was normal, but she didn't feel any love for him.

In contrast, her father's parents were wealthy, and they lived in a large house. Mrs. O. spent all her vacations with them, and the strictest punishment for her was when her mother forbade her to go to them. When her father visited his parents and took her out for dinner, those were the best memories from her childhood. She felt cozy there and never wanted to return to her mother's house. Mrs. O. especially remembers herself at the age of 8–10 when she longed for her father. Her paternal grandmother understood this; she often played dolls with the analysand, and in her later years, she took her to restaurants to teach her good manners and taught her how to dress and walk with good posture. However, according to Mrs. O., all of this was associated with the fact that her grandparents perceived her as a poor child with a bad upbringing and a lack of manners. The analysand always wanted to prove to them that she was worthy and wanted them to be proud of her because she felt like a second-class one.

After school, Mrs. O. wanted to become a lawyer like her father, but her mother and paternal grandfather decided that it would be better for her to enroll in medical university. In her final year, she wanted to choose a specialization like her mother, who was a midwife, but after practice, she decided to choose a dermatological specialization. During university, she fell in love with a guy. He had just had an argument with his girlfriend and started dating Mrs. O. He became her first sexual partner – their relationship continued for over half a year, until one day he informed her that he had decided to return to his previous girlfriend. Soon after, he married that girl. Her name was the same as the girl who was born to her father from another marriage. But their communication didn't end, transitioning into a friendship. Mr. S. called almost daily, and when his son was born, he even left the child with Mrs. O., secretly from his wife. Meanwhile, to spite him, Mrs. O. began dating his friend, who was studying to be a soldier. Very soon, she got married, and when Mr. S. found out about it, he ceased all communication with her.

Mrs. O. never loved her husband; their sexual relations didn't satisfy her, but she thought she could build a normal family if she was wise. She directed a significant amount of energy into building her business projects and making money, and she succeeded in it. Mr. S. often appeared in her dreams; she maintained a Facebook page with one goal – for him to see that everything was going well for her and regret leaving her. She said it was all like fantasies she lived with normally, and everything would have continued like that if not for the war.

Mrs. O.'s husband was a military man, so he was immediately mobilized for service in the Ukrainian armed forces; he came home every weekend. In the spring of 2023, due to certain circumstances, after 13 years, Mrs. O. starts communicating with Mr. S. They develop romantic relations, and soon everyone finds out about it, and a big scandal erupts in both families. For a while, the scandal subsides, but the romantic relationship continues. At some point, Mrs. O. realizes that these relationships have no future, and that Mr. S. is not whom she fantasized about, but for some reason, she couldn't end the relationship.

Each clinical case inevitably faces us with the repetition of part of the story or traumatic event that the patient unconsciously reenacts in the therapist's office. This is to symbolize what remains unprocessed, forgotten, and repressed, but resurfaces in symptoms or other forms of suffering, in fantasies or dreams, prompting patients to seek help from a psychoanalyst. Reflecting on this case, one might assume that Mrs. O. sought therapy for the first time, choosing an analyst with the same name as both her rivals: her sister, born of her father's second marriage, and Mr. S.'s wife. In couples therapy, she seemed to recreate the situation where she competed for the man who belonged to her rival. After completing couples therapy and working individually, she acknowledged that not all women with that name were bad and reflected on how her attitude toward the analyst related to her history. Her sudden desire to end therapy due to moving to another city resembled a childhood dream of permanently moving to the wealthy home of her paternal family. However, why she confided her greatest secret to the analyst remained unexplained at the time.

This became clear when Mrs. O. returned to therapy during the war. She said that Mr. S. attracted her during their student years because he resembled her father – intelligent and unattainable. During times when they didn't communicate, she maintained social media pages to make Mr. S. regret not choosing her. This closely resembled her childhood dream where her father would choose her over her sister, with whom she always competed and tried to surpass. Mrs. O. also admitted that now she allows herself to play with Mr. S. in the literal sense of the word, explaining it as something she didn't get to do in childhood. Her father was the only one who played with her, bought her toys, and spent time with her. She hardly remembered herself before the age of six, and this forgetting was related to her mother not allowing her father to visit her until she was six and throwing away the toys he sent for her.

Thus, after Mrs. O.'s return, the therapist came to the following conclusion. When in previous therapy, the patient approached her repressed feelings toward her father and mother, her confession about living with her husband while loving Mrs. O. seemed to legalize her hatred toward her mother and rivalry with her for her father's love.

It is notable how the war influenced the romantic side of Mrs. O.'s life. Reflecting on this, one might assume that the war allowed her to once again feel how important her father was in her life and allowed her to enter into a relationship with a married man. Despite her mother's prohibition, she played with the toys her father gave her. When the war began and the patient's husband started coming home only on weekends, it seemed to bring her back to childhood, where her stepfather also came on weekends, and she never had her place: neither in her father's family nor in her own, where she didn't even have her bed, reinforcing those unprocessed feelings of sorrow and suffering for her father. These experiences awakened infantile desires that had been protected under repression.

During one session, Mrs. O. pondered: "Why do they love some, but marry others," evidently reflecting that the image of the man in her psychic reality is split into the stepfather, whom she didn't love and was forced to live with, and the father, whom she loved but belonged to another woman. In other words, she is replaying the life script of her childhood. She lives in two families: one where she feels bad but is forced to live with her husband and the other where she feels good but is not accepted because her lover has his own family. Emotional regression brought her back to the times when her father was the best man in the world for her, the embodiment of all her dreams. In the therapist's office, there was a girl who had gone through her Oedipus complex, rejected incestuous desires toward her father, but still felt aggression toward her mother and believed she could find someone just like her father.

The war intensified the sense of death, so seeking new romantic relationships, and trying to revive old love affairs, is one manifestation of the drive for life, for self-preservation. "It's better to do it today because there's no certainty about tomorrow," said Mrs. O., explaining her infidelity to her husband.

Now, the focus of our work is on what Freud (1924) termed the dissolution of the Oedipus complex, the destruction of the phallic organization. Rejecting one's childhood perception of the parental couple as omnipotent beings, reinterpreting childhood history as a result, and the ability to have a realistic view of those who are close – all these are tasks of adolescent development. It appears that Mrs. O. is mentally approaching the realization that no love can be eternal.

Beginning of October 2023 (1 Year 8 Months into the War)

"My soul is bigger than my body" – is the direct quote from the patient.

A woman of striking appearance entered the office – quite revealing attire, high heels, jewelry, and long well-groomed hair. She looked too glamorous and attractive, not typical for everyday life. It immediately struck me as reminiscent of how liberated girls looked in the 90s.

Mrs. A. was 42 years old, divorced in 2010, with a daughter with a severe disability. She boasted that she was currently earning well, that she had overcome the "sick child complex," that she had always been a beautiful and smart girl, and graduated from school with honors. She now lives with her mother, who helps take care of her sick daughter at home, where her parents have lived all their lives.

She complained about her personal life. She said she had a very difficult year, that she had lived alone for a long time, that is, without a husband ("lived" was spoken in the past tense, as if she was not living alone now). She said she couldn't figure out her self-esteem because on the one hand, she's so perfect that it's scary to get close to her, and on the other hand, the guys she likes don't like her, probably because she's too honest. She noted that she doesn't know her worth (I assumed Mrs. A. was talking about her value to someone). And most importantly, she is troubled by the fact that she wants to forget the man she fought with at the end of May 2023.

Family Story of Mrs. A.

The father of Mrs. A. came from a poor rural family, which belonged to the local intelligentsia. His father was a teacher of the German language, and his mother was a teacher of elementary classes. After finishing school, Mrs. A.'s father entered the institute at the faculty of physical education in the city where the examinee's mother lived. They met and got married, and began living in the house of Mrs. A.'s mother's parents (the same house where she currently resides). They had three daughters, and Mrs. A. was the middle one.

When Mrs. A. was 5 years old, her parents along with their daughters moved abroad, as her father was offered a job as a sports instructor. Later, there was a scandalous incident at her father's workplace, where some girl accused him of harassment, and the whole family had to return to Ukraine. The analysand said, "Father was difficult because he cheated on mom, but he didn't abandon us."

Mrs. A. recounted that her father was the best man among her surroundings. She described her father quite warmly, portraying him as a good, tidy, strong, athletic man who was a pillar of support for the family, earning enough money to ensure his daughters were always well-dressed. He wanted a son, so he called his daughters his "Cossacks" (Cossacks – free armed people, representatives of the military estate, mercenaries. Members of self-governing male military communities that existed in the territories of the Ukrainian "Wild Field" from the 15th century, in the region between the middle reaches of the Dnipro and Don rivers, at the border of the Christian and Muslim worlds. In Ukrainian, "Cossack" is a masculine noun). He taught his daughters to fight and defend themselves. The analysand recalled that they always felt protected; for example, she mentioned an incident in the 90s when there was a group of boys – gangsters who raped girls, in the area where they lived. The father threatened these boys so that they wouldn't dare to touch his daughters. The sisters didn't like Mrs. A, they called her arrogant and unapproachable, because she acted like a "Queen" and never backed down. Also, she was mom's favorite, and of all the sisters, she was the closest to her. The patient started a sexual life when she was 14, and when she was 15, she secretly had an abortion. She was sexually active, she frequently changed partners. Once, her father told her that it was unacceptable: if she was seeing a guy, she should only stay with him, "if with one, then with one."

The father suddenly passed away at the age of 42, in early October. Mrs. A. was 19 years old at the time. She remembers her bewilderment at the funeral, wondering how her father could lie in the ground. After his death, the family's financial situation worsened significantly, as her mother had never worked anywhere. At that time, she was studying at the institute and was involved with a guy. She became pregnant at the age of 20 and she had an abortion on her mother's demand.

She still regrets it to this day. Mrs. A. broke up with that guy under her mother's pressure and started dating another one who, according to her mother, was promising and from a good family. They got married, and they had a daughter. When the child was almost 3 years old, she was diagnosed with a severe form of autism. Her relationship with her husband deteriorated, and when their daughter was 5 years old, Mrs. A. moved back in with her mother. Eventually, she divorced her husband. She then had two more attempts to establish relationships with men, but these men were not what she desired.

Before the war, Mrs. A. had gone 9 years without any romantic or sexual relationships. She worked a lot, and it seemed that at that time she was content with compliments on her photos on social media. The war caught her off guard. The house she lives in is near a military airfield that was bombed on the first day of the war. For a long time, she, her disabled daughter, her mother, and her grandmother lived in the basement. She recalls feeling helpless, unprotected, and frozen as if life had come to an end. A few weeks later, a guy from another country wrote to her on Instagram: "How are you?" She noticed that this guy had written to her before, but she hadn't paid attention to him. However, she replied that they survived the rocket attack. He responded: "Come to me, I'll help as much as possible."

After those words, something inside her changed, she began to fantasize about the man she had been waiting for all her life. He embodied all her preferences: he was handsome, and athletic, and told her that he had a prestigious profession. She sincerely told him her story about her disabled child and how she was coping well with it because she earned enough to support her family. She felt that he understood her. She also believed that if there were mass rocket attacks, she could go to him with her child. She remembered that she had once dreamed of living in this country because it was sunny and had the sea. They began a romantic correspondence for almost a year. During this time, she felt protected, as she once did when her father was alive.

"The war stirred me up and brought me back to life," Mrs. A. said at one of the sessions. She often dreamed of her father. In her dreams, he was alive, and she was very happy about it. In March 2023, she bought tickets with her own money and went on a trip for the first time in 9 years. She flew to the man of her dreams who lived in the country of her childhood fantasies. But in reality, everything turned out differently from her dreams. She liked the guy, "he even had the same stubble as her father."

But it seemed that he was not looking for a relationship but a wealthy sponsor. In May of the same year, they argued.

At the beginning of October, she went to therapy. It was the anniversary of her father's death, and she had just reached the age at which her father died. She complained that she couldn't forget a man she had fallen in love with. In one of the sessions, she said,

> It's hard to let go of a dream. My father has been gone for twenty-three years now, but he still appears in my dreams, as if he came back to life and we treat him very carefully. I had a dream yesterday that I was swimming in the pool with my father, and a child was with us. My father's slipper falls to the very bottom, he wants to dive after it, but I say he shouldn't, that he has high blood pressure. I see the slipper sinking to the bottom, lying among the algae. I look at my father and rejoice that he has come back to life; I don't want him to die again. He shouldn't strain himself; I want to protect him.

Reflecting on this case, one might assume that feelings of helplessness and fear of war triggered the need for a strong parental figure that would make her feel protected. Along with dreams of protection from her father, feelings of her childhood were also triggered. Mrs. A. fondly remembered her father, seemingly ignoring his misdeeds. The image of her father remained highly idealized: "My father is the best man in my surroundings."

It seemed that after losing her father, she became a little girl again, seeking security and returning to her mother's favorite child. Perhaps it is precisely because she still sees herself as a child that she says, "My soul is bigger than my body." The little body belongs to a girl, not a woman, and a girl can only give birth to children in fantasies. After divorcing her husband, she refrains from romantic and sexual relationships for many years.

It can be assumed that this is like fulfilling the parental commandment to be only with one man. In her story, this means being faithful to her deceased father.

When a guy from Instagram asked her, "How are you?" it revived her infantile fantasies, and she felt valuable to someone other than her mother again. Mrs. A. noted that it stirred her up and revived her. She began to have more dreams in which her father came back to life, and she worried that he might die again.

It is also worth noting that during this period, the relationship with her mother deteriorated significantly. Mrs. A. did not understand why her mother criticized her because her mother often started saying that she looked like a prostitute. In the first sessions, she made an impression of being a rather vulgar person. Her clothing was indeed similar to what prostitutes usually wear. This presentation sharply contrasted with the fact that in reality, she had been lonely for many years.

At one of the sessions, Mrs. A. said that for the first time in many years, she wants to have meaningful relationships with a worthy man and create a family with him, wanting to "rediscover her femininity." Her style of dressing has also changed. Lately, she wears clothing of white or black monocolor, in which she looks either like a bride or like a widow.

Conclusion

Based on our clinical observations, we can state that a person feels the tyranny of time most acutely during wartime, and similarly, one can keenly feel the interconnectedness of life and death during such times. If at the beginning of the war the expression "if it weren't for the war, this would never have happened" from our patients meant losses, destruction, and death, then 12 months from the start of the war, they used the same words to talk about new romantic relationships and betrayals. The fear of death can lead a person to perceive life as a permit to do something new. We are accustomed to the notion that war arouses a desire for death because it is death itself. However, just as there is no death without life, there is no war without a desire for self-preservation.

Studying stories of love and betrayal during wartime, we always consider the influence of the infantile object, childhood fantasies, and the passage of the Oedipal conflict on a person's subsequent erotic life. This chapter focuses on the stories of two women, but we observe similar processes to some extent in the lives of our male patients as well. The Oedipus complex is the basis for structuring personality, the transition from life in the dimension of demand to the dimension of desire.

In his paper "*Autobiography*," Freud (2013) stated that along with understanding how widespread the Oedipus complex is, he also came to realize that through it, the path to the regularities of the mental process in its affective significance is revealed. In a letter to Fliess Freud (1897) shared that he understood the power with which the myth of King Oedipus captivated the viewer or reader. This fascination happens because the Greek myth reveals an intrusive impulse that every person recognizes by tracing it within themselves.

References

Freud, S. (1955). Analysis of a phobia in a five-year-old boy. *Collected Papers*, 3, 149–289.

Freud, S. (1961). The infantile genital organization (an interpolation into the theory of sexuality). In *The standard edition of the complete psychological works of Sigmund Freud, Volume XIX: The Ego and the Id and Other Works (1923–1925)* (pp. 139–146). London: Hogarth Press.

Freud, S. (2013). *The autobiography of Sigmund Freud.* Read Books Ltd.

Freud, S., & Strachey, J. (1955). *Beyond the pleasure principle* (Vol. 18, pp. 3–64). Hogarth Press.

Freud, S., & Strachey, J. (1986). Three essays on the theory of sexuality: I: The sexual aberrations. In M. Buckley (Ed.) *Essential Papers on Object Relations* (pp. 5–39). New York University Press.

Freud, S., & Strachey, J. (2001). *A case of hysteria, three essays on sexuality, and other works* (Vol. 7). Random House.

Lacan, J. (2011). *The seminar of Jacques Lacan: Book V: The formations of the unconscious: 1957–1958.* Eres.

Laplanche, J., & Pontalis, J. B. (2018). *The language of psychoanalysis.* Routledge.

Pavlovska, O. (2024). Experiencing time: The subject between destructive and constructive processes. *Ukrainian Psychoanalytic Journal*, 2(1), 8–13. https://doi.org/10.32782/upj/2024-1-2.

Yevlanova, E. (2023). Professional supervision as therapist' self-care during wartime. *Psychoanalytic Psychology*, 40(4), 257.

Chapter 4

"I Do (Not) Want to Kill": Trauma Beyond Words

Olena Medvedieva

From Silence to Cry

Typically, despite the recognition that we should embrace silence, which stands in opposition to our loud routines, we feel the terror caused by silence. We tend to be cautious. Silence is not an absence of noise. We associate silence with an experience of an abandoned ancient church, or with the silence of the bottom of a well, or with one of lovers holding their breath. There is also the silence of cold hallways of metro stations and bomb shelters, those undergrounds and basements that hide confused people during the bombings. During the first weeks of war, I would dedicate a few hours to go there and try to talk to the terrified people, urging them to articulate words. The words were lacking. People not only could not talk but also could not change their clothes, wash, eat or sleep. People cried a lot. Tears are also types of words that cannot be articulated. The silence was total and intrusive, as it pushed toward shelters even without air raid sirens. People often reported having sound hallucinations, which occurred especially in the silence of night. When the darkness is torn by the sound of sirens, as the sound resonance is enhanced, hearing becomes the main feeling function at night. It reminded me of the Barthelemy's (1997) description of the silence in a desert that isn't merely an opposite to noise but is a state that takes a person to a different dimension of reality and thus immediately becomes a part of the inner world and therefore creates a new link to reality. The ability to suffer silently is often presented as a virtue. However, psychoanalysts hold a different opinion: speak, we say, so that I can hear you. This notion was also held by Socrates. During the war, we Ukrainians realized that silence can also speak.

Corbin (2018) in *A History of Silence* provided an example of contrast between silence and acoustic hell, which can hold huge sound clutter, clang

DOI: 10.4324/9781032660257-5

of weapons, cries of anger and suffering, and rattling breath of those who die at war. Learning to distinguish the noise and silence is required of those who want to survive, as you should listen to the devastating silence of a bullet that aims in your direction. Corbin notes that in wartime, silence follows the death toll of someone dying and being mourned for. Silence speaks toward the fear of death, as cemeteries are silent, interrupted only by the cries. It's similar to Mallarmé's (2011) description of the silence of death, which is miserly and long like the night and only takes meanings for the living. This understanding depicts the silence that was common not only in bomb shelters but also during our individual sessions when our analysands needed time to even be able to physically speak. They would often begin with either whisper or crying, and only then be able to form words. Whisper is like a distant cry: it is the quiver of voice and the flesh that precedes any sound.

Is crying a form of speech? The causes of crying are pain, frustration, anxiety. And the moment the Other hears and becomes the addressee, when the Other answers, the cry turns into a call retroactively as it becomes interpreted. The cry acquires a meaning and the first function of speech, which is to address to the Other and gain a response from them. Freud (1920/2015) in his *Beyond the Pleasure Principle* considers the birth of a subject: a baby separated from itself as a result of discharge of emotional suffering due to the interruption of homeostasis. The discharge of the inner pressure takes a form of cry. The acoustic self-expression acts as evacuation of pressure. This cry is not futile though, as it attracts the attention of the caretaker, performs a specific act to neutralize the suffering. The cry constitutes into a call in response to the voice of the Other that signifies a wish aimed at the child. The power of drive makes the baby produce voice to find the Other and get a response from them. Thus, having read the resonance in the tune of the Other, the subject starts to accept it and eliminate it as a call for approaching and moving away when the subject becomes deaf to his own voice. This process lets the voice take its place. Mother will interpret the cry as a foreseen articulation from the baby. She has to accept this cry, assuming the baby wants to say something, which means that something that represents the subject for the Other takes place. The cry does not represent the child to mother, and in this case, we are in the register of the sign. It represents, first of all, the subject to everyone who will come in the future. The response of the Other means that they leave some space to accept the "pure cry" which they turn into a "cry for something." A cry caused by need turns into a demand that outreaches the need, as it is a call that requires attention and reaction.

Cries and moans have become the expression of a call to the Other of psychoanalyst during war, the one who can hear and interpret it because they are in the same frame of war, pain, and sufferings. When people lacked for words to express trauma, they cried and expressed it through tears. A woman who came to analysis two months after the war began could only cry and moan quietly. She lost her husband. For her the time had stopped, and she lacked words to describe her pain. It lasted until the voice appeared in the frame of the room as a safe space with the Other present and listening.

Should psychoanalysts break the silence? Noticeably, in these situations, it is important to not just cover the temporary breach in the symbolic. On the contrary, it makes sense to leave the trauma non-symbolized for some time as a gap that may let something true and important for the subject squeeze in. The moving boundary will then open its territories. This process means that insisting and facilitating articulation of the traumatic material to make analysand feel better immediately is an absolutely wrong idea. When we talk about the trauma of subject, we think about it through this circle of repetition. It remains fixed as it cannot acquire a meaning that would make the being of subject integrated, acquisitive of evolution, and as it does not let symbolization happen. Thus, it has the tendency to repeat as it is. Long fixations on traumas cause mental and somatic symptoms due to exhaustion of our psyche in its attempts to prevent the repetition of traumatic experience. The object freezes any way of activation. The analyst's job is then to help the patient integrate the past in the conditions of enough safety, overcoming the pressure of return, gradually ruining the counter-measures the patient uses to avoid the return of trauma. Subject develops new experience in analysis. Something that has already been said in analysis may change its meaning in the light of the new movement. An analytical session can then become the space that connects the past, present, and future.

Following the logic of structural psychoanalysis, Lacan (1973–1974/2011) suggested that analysts view psychic phenomena as an intersection of the Symbolic, the Imaginary, and the Real (i.e., third topica). The Symbolic is a set of differentiated, separate elements called signifiers. The Real is the most concealed part of the psyche that always slips away from imagination and word description. The Real of the psyche is so incomprehensible that Lacan uses Kant's "thing-in-itself" to characterize it. The Imaginary is an individual way of perceiving the symbolic order, a person's subjective image of the world and own self, first of all. The Real is connected with the body, birth, death, and speechlessness. Thus, the Real is what gets rejected from subjective meaning, what every subject considers impossible. When the war started, shock was the first reaction. How can one believe that airports are bombed, tanks crush cars, the enemy tortures and murders children, houses burn, or women are raped? Indeed, the invasion into the country was perceived as an invasion into the body of every Ukrainian person. This is the moment when we face the Real. The Symbolic enters in to it. Psychoanalysts know that the process of facing the Real takes place through verbal impotence, through physical suffering that people bear deep in their flesh. That is why we deal with the Real but cannot say anything about it. Analytical constructs work when they reconstruct our attitude toward the Real. This is what is indeed significant. This is the reason why Ukrainian psychoanalysts could not stay silent during the war. We worked, so that our people would get an ability to speak.

Lacan would also ask what makes people enter psychoanalysis, attributing this choice to something becoming unbearable due to the invasion of the Real and this something slipping away from people and making them too anxious, only being able to imagine how the Real crushes them, or – even more specifically – strangulates them and cuts of their air.

Psychoanalysis is the only means that can let us go through the Real. Trauma and subjective structure are our fundamental phantasm. They are interconnected, and it is important to understand not what damaged us but why it damaged us, which gives an event the traumatic value. According to Medvedieva (2024):

> That is because the historization of the past is seen as the essence and basis of analysis while the goal of therapy in psychoanalytical approach is then to let analysands see themselves not as absent, frozen, distant, excluded, but as the witnesses of historical events. This will let them gradually find the parts of their souls that were left in the past and think toward the future through painful experience. Because in general, social tragedies, wars – long, past or recent – will long stand out with bright flashes of memories, dark spots of inhibition, black holes of losses, transparent freezes with different rhythms, leaving inevitable traces in individual history.
>
> (pp. 32–44)

Lacan (1953–1954/1999) in his *Les Écrits Techniques de Freud, Séminaire* believed that traumatic meaning doesn't always follow the event, which triggered it. Instead this meaning moves to the category of non-repressed unconscious, something that hasn't been integrated into the verbalized system of the person and therefore hasn't achieved meaning. These events then resurface in memory by becoming articulated as the subject goes further into the more organized symbolic world. These memories keep intruding and reoccur. Thus, trauma is an insignificant experience, it doesn't predefine or precedes the symptom. This experience constitutes on the basis of retrospective influence of the second scene on the first one, constituting the first scene as repressed one based on the general signifiers.

Moreover, the mental structure as suggested by Lacan (1968) *The Language of the Self: The Function of Language in Psychoanalysis* is inevitably composed in every person as an effect of birth of the Other subject, language, and culture. As mental structure appears as a result of birth of a "creature that speaks," in its course of constitutive estrangement into language as the house of being. The third one in the psychoanalyst's room is the Other speech, and speech is the main sign of structure. The grand Other is a symbolic order to the extent with which it particularizes for every separate subject. The Other is this another subject in its radical otherness and uniqueness that cannot be assimilated, but is at the same time a symbolic order that mediates in our relationship with another subject. The Other should be mostly understood as space – a space where speech is created. Stating that speech is born in the other, Lacan (1957/2011) noted that language and speech are beyond our conscious control. They come from beyond consciousness, hence unconscious being the discourse of the Other. In his concept of viewing the Other as space, Lacan dwells upon Freud's mental topica that describes the unconscious as "a different place."

Language is a mediator between thought and sound. Language is what expresses thinking, thought, through the sound of voice. Speech sign is a mental image acquired from sound, understanding and acoustic image. Therefore, a signifier is an understanding, a thing, an action. Signified is an acoustic image. The variety of human relationships is described by Lacan's (1972–1973/2011) sophisticated aphorism: "Signifier represents the subject to another signifier" (p. 43) The point of this phrase is that a person uses language in communication to let the Other know what they are and what they want, which can only be carried out through the words of language (that signify). The signified is the person themselves, their Ego. This process also concerns the colloquist, the Other, who additionally represents himself with the help of words. Signifiers, connected into a chain, are subject to the double movement of connecting metonymy and displacement – a metaphor. This movement defines the structure, moving one of the elements into the periphery, while the unoccupied space is called deficiency.

Thus, at the same time, while traumatic scene is articulated as "enigmatic signifier," repressed signifier, the symptom produces an effect of metaphorical meaning, the haste of synchronic interruption in current sequence. In those sufferings, guilt is attributed to the past, shame to the present, and the so-called concern to the future. Guilt is about the decision made and carried out in the past. Shame is felt as a loss of safety, while concern turns out to be obsessive about decisive moments in the future. A subject complains in the present. The actual symptom chronicles the "virtual signifier" of trauma without creating a general dimension. A subject can be attached to consequences of events throughout the entire life.

Ferrell (2006) suggested, using Freud's theory, that being heard meets the expression of the cry. This active position will only be perceived after an action as a result of meeting the Other that will make this call heard while the Other will transform it into an acoustic eruption, a vocal manifestation of the state of helplessness, an inquiry, and then one should achieve subject's ability to speak. The subject then produces voice that looks for the ear of the Other to get a response, as noted by Vivès (2013). The person is engaged into speech, called by origin, and structures in oneself is the not deaf and able to hear Other, thus becoming the one who calls. In this situation, the person captures his own voice and as if starts hearing himself. The subject does not talk to the Other but with the power of his voice calls to the Other, as subject's voice has the power to call to himself as well as to those who can hear him. We had to hear and say: You are not alone. As for a psychoanalyst it means he or she should specifically "attach" themselves to the sufferings of those who come to see them. Psychoanalyst is certainly less free than any other person in this matter.

From Voice to Word

The voices of war are ambivalent. There is one that supports the moral law, and there are voice of mind, voice of heart, calling voice, avenging voice, voice of pain. It seems that humanity generally is of a vocal nature, and in times of challenges, vocality changes its score. As voice is always connected with the compelling presence of the Other. Voice is the carrier of speech, the basis of word, sentence, discourse of expression. Voice is something special with the background of acoustic phenomena, as it has an inner connection with meaning. As only voice foresees subjectivity that expresses itself. Voice makes an expression possible, however it disappears in it like a mirage, in a meaning that is produced, and after all becomes the object that connects the subject and the Other that does not turn into smoke during the meaning. Hence, at the beginning of psychoanalysis, there was voice.

Voice proceeds before word and makes the understanding of it possible. Moreover, while the word grows, voices recede. Voice is an attempt to convince the Other to listen. It penetrates the inner, discloses it, and the outer becomes uncertain without it. There are many voices in the outside. At the same time, the voice that comes from the inside brings more than what we intend to say, while also different. Freud (1899/2022) believed that dream interpretation takes an analyst on a road of discovering the unconscious with Lacan (1968) further suggesting that the unconscious is structured like speech. A Slovenian psychoanalyst Dolar (2006) expanded Lacan's statement by coining the term "excrescence," which means that the Voice, albeit being the King's highway, doesn't speak on its own. Voice is a tool, a way, a means, and meaning is the goal. Voice is a material element. It is present in the act of speech but is nevertheless elusive, non-linguistic. However, voice is individual, subjective, similar to fingerprints, can be identified instantly. Voice in the formations of unconscious is nothing but its formation that is connected with drive, fantasy, and wish. If the unconscious can be described, it is only because it speaks. Freud (1905) separated the life and death drives, they could also be viewed as related to voice, as the noise of life is Eros, and the mysterious Thanatos is silent. Both drives are of course interconnected, and the silence of the death drive accompanies the noise of life.

The history of voice in psychoanalysis is fascinating – it was at the beginning of psychoanalysis and still accompanies it. However, to dispose of one's own voice, a child should avoid admiring the voice of the Other. Lippi (2014), using Vivès' ideas, suggested that the subject requires to have an intrapsychic point. It is the point of deafness in which the subject becomes deaf to be able to master his own voice. The visual dimension is structured by absence, while the acoustic field is constructed around the point of deafness. We can avert our gaze but we cannot avert our ears. One cannot avoid the voice of the Other. The hypothesis about the point of deafness lets us think about the development of subject in the acoustic field and the way the subject creates own relationship with the voice of the Other. This is the example of an act between analyst and analysand. Because what is important is not the words that act but the subjective position that supports the words. Thus, the subject may become capable of responding to Other's demand affirmatively: "Become it!" The caring environment can be represented by the psychoanalyst. At the moment of analytical meeting, the voice will "stupefy" and thus establish a wish. To understand this, we need to be able to differentiate between two voices. The first one is silent and is purely a call to what is supposed to take place – it foreshadows the coming of the Real. The second voice is in speech that puts reality that happens into a form.

Voice is between body and speech but doesn't belong to them. Any drive that is placed outside the body is an extension of the body. Drives are not outside though, they are on the verge. Voice is also in the junction of speech and body, is common, comes from body but is not its part. It supports speech but does not belong to it. The subject is forever stuck between the voice and understanding, captured in the temporality of fantasy and desire. Hence, first we have a voice-object, and then the signifiers as a way to understand, reconcile with the voice. The intimacy that voice comes from is described by Freud as uncanny, it is a call from the uncanny. Certainly, the most uncanny for human beings is death, or a dead body. Freud (1919/2017) in the *Uncanny* prepares the grounds for his future theory of life and death drives. In the *Uncanny*, one can see the transition from Freud's early thoughts about denial of death and the ruination of this denial by the topic of war to the new idea about life that strives for death, that is a central thought of *Beyond the Pleasure Principle*.

Loraux (2002), a historian and Hellenist, in her study entitled *The Mourning Voice* transformed our understanding of the Greek tragedy. She invited the reader to move beyond the political dimension that is usually put forward in the tragic literature and hear the real human voice that is expressed in a complaint more vocalized than articulated. Ayay is a dreary word without meaning in which the sound prevails over the meaning – the hero says it when facing the tragic. The tragedy then is a place not only for word but mostly for voice. The voice here is touching and lets the viewer be seized by the transmitted message. Essentially, that's how an analyst know the psychoanalysis is happening: The subject not only produces voice, the person is also produced by it. Indeed, there is no subject without a call that invites him to exist. There is no subject without a call enforced by voice. On this basis, psychoanalysis lets us think about paradoxically ambivalent connection that exists between subject and voices that surround the person – necessary and at the same time invasive – thus we can offer the renewed analysis of social mechanisms aimed at finding the voice and keeping it at a distance.

Slovenian psychoanalyst M. Dolar (2006) expanded the topic by labeling the voice as the somatic basis of speech; it acts irrespectively of the modality of feelings that express it. This means that voice is the body part that needs to be activated, metaphorically sacrificed, in order to create a statement. Thus, the voice disappears behind the meaning as the basis of discourse expression. Freud (1937/1959) in *Analysis Terminable and Interminable* discussed three impossible professions that are impossible because we will always be unhappy with the results – government, education, and psychoanalysis. All three have voice at their cores. Moreover, perhaps that is the element that makes them impossible. They are impossible because they deal with transference, and voice functions as a lever of transfer, and perhaps transference is putting letters into action with the help of voice. Psychoanalysis can be only carried out with live voice and not recorded. Analysand vocalizes associations that come to mind in the presence of analyst, and he or she is basically the only speaker. Analyst should more often be silent while it makes sense. However, everything is contrarily here: Analyst becomes the embodiment of voice as object, a personification, embodied voice, not the voice of Super-Ego but the impossible voice that requires a response. The voice that does not say anything, the voice of the urge to answer, meaning it adopts the own position as a subject. It is urged to say what comes to mind to break the silence, and the entire analysis becomes a way to learn to take over the voice. That is why at the beginning of psychoanalysis there was voice. Voice goes before word and makes the understanding of it possible. The word will have sense, proposing a sound to ears, proposing something to mind. Additionally, while the word grows, voices recede.

From Word to Speech

When something falls out of the Symbolic and Imaginary and slips away from the imaginary confrontation, Lacan (1957) calls it a-object which, while being real, is something lost, something that has been defeated. Thus, it interests us exactly because it poses a challenge. It is the reason of wish. This object becomes the object of phantasm, meaning something that seizes us from outside and also belongs to us as well as is an object of drives. The list of a-objects includes such valuables as voice, breast, gaze, genitals, and such unpleasant ones as feces. Assuming we have no words to express what we feel toward the enemy, how painful, anxious, frightening it is, how scared we are of losing the body, meaning life, we can still "talk in a specific way." Using the common language of drives, we overcome traumas with the help of connecting valuable organs – penis and vagina – with anal objects, and what cannot be expressed is then used as curses: "fuck russia," "fucking orc," "russian warship, go fuck yourself," and so forth. The object in two instances – imaginary and real – then has a double value: disgust and desire, as abusive language is not just one sense, and generally it urges to articulate the trauma.

One of the fundamental principles pointed out by Lacan (1966) was that the structure of the unconscious is similar to language, or, similarly, that the unconscious is knowledge structured like language. We are the creatures that have language, and we are the creatures that language lives in. We are creatures outclassed by language, the word is ahead of us and astounds us. That means that language lives in us beyond analysis, and we always feel its influence. We are creatures in which the signified takes a form of speech, it gets articulated independently of us.

The unconscious is structured like language. However, its effects exist with the background of speech. The symbolic system in which subject exists is indeed complicated. Subjects are not just participants of a symbolic field, but more those who experience the influence of speech symbols as universum. The goal of the subject then is to find its place in the general language. In psychoanalytical act, speech is a consent between two subjects that includes the attempt to solve or sometimes cut the knots of speech. Furthermore, the symbolic system is complicated, and in order to disentangle it and find the truth, one needs to demystify these subjective camouflages – that is what psychoanalytical method means, according to Lacan. In psychoanalytical discourse we carefully keep track of the moments when language controls speech, but it as if slips out of our control, like for instance a dream or symptom. This is what we call psychoanalytical experience. As Hanna Segal (2006) suggested, when the world inside us is destroyed, when it is dead and gets no love, when our closest people are fragmented, and we are helplessly desperate, we have to recreate our world, combine the parts, bring life to dead fragments, and recreate life.

War has become a common symptom. Sufferings are expressed through a specific language, they create new frames of linguistic dimension, because subject always connects his sufferings with own interpretation, explains the reasons with the ways of own experience, comes to therapy with an own version, but the unconscious is expressed in speech through the filter of conscious. Today we hear that war has raised and affected something in the subjective dimension that is personal, repressed, but its articulation has become possible with the help of circumstances that pushed into articulation of the collective trauma.

Analysand X. came to therapy as he had become as if deaf for some time, then was unable to speak. The affect happened in his bathroom when he caught the text on some old bottles of cream that belonged to his girlfriend. It said "Made in Russia." The bottles were swept from the shelf but he does not remember what happened next. The voice in his head said: "Full-scale invasion." He wailed, cried, then froze and forgot words. It happened in early autumn, the war went on already. The man would come at assigned time, sit in the armchair in front of me and remain silent. That lasted for several days. I also kept silent, creating the safest space of frame. The first phrase he said was: "I want to kill rusnia (Russians, neglectful)." The symptom has two sides: sign and signifier. The sign is connected with assumption. Some event happens, analysand explains it, puts analyst in the position of the Other of this symptom and its reasons – that is basically how psychoanalysis works. Lacanian (1972–1973/2011) idea of a sign is something that represents something to somebody. That means it is something important for the subject and for the one who listens, meaning the analyst. Thus, this is something that favors transference, and psychoanalysts today become included into the speech frames of war, although what analysand talks about is intersubjective.

At the session when he was able to talk, he said he wanted to go to the army, so that he would be sent to kill "rusnia." Analysand came with a shoulder bag that had a first aid kit in it, according to him. It was interesting: He was going to kill and took a first aid kit with him – to help whom? The answer-denial: "Rusnia are not people" made him think: I need to save those I want to kill. I do (not) want to kill. X. has a strong Russian accent in his speech. He used a lot of Russian words but tried to speak Ukrainian. He comes from Zaporizhzhia, a city with many Russian-speaking Ukrainians. His parents still live there. "When did you start speaking Ukrainian?" "I wanted in 2014 but didn't, so I started in February 2024, when the war started." He called father in the morning. Father answered him in Russian, just as before. Analysand said he did not reproach him, although he wanted to. But since then, he started to feel the aggression growing in him, and it was harder to control it every following day. The trauma of war is an especially dramatic example as we feel that the world strives to get us, that is "they try to kill me." In Klein's (1987) logic, the extent of trauma mostly depends on how reliably the traumatized person is in a depressive position in which they take the responsibility for their own aggression and hatred. These feelings are the real source of trauma. Moreover, subject has them toward previously good objects as well. He is afraid so that he would not be able to protect them from his own rage. Trauma strengthens the paranoid-schizoid experience of reality that is always present, has always strived to be heard but was subject to depressive experience, by which Klein (1987) means orientation at care and responsibility for the world or one's own small part of it. Since the beginning of war, X. has not felt anxiety, as he says, because as one of the heads of company he would responsibly organize the evacuation of other employees, cared about others, was "the senior one." It was interesting, because the importance of those who recognized him and the desperation of his looking for those objects also made me think about his father.

The man recalled the period when the family lived in Israel. He was cruelly beaten in a multinational school, "even broke my arm because I was Russian, they called me that." He complained to father, asked for protection, at least explanation and support, but father said he should be proud of the fact he was Russian. Back there, in Israel, patient found a senior student who taught him to fight back. But when he fought, it was hard to control aggression: "Perhaps I tried to kill rusnia already then, in myself" The actual trauma of war raised the Oedipal trauma. Father only recognized his elder son. He mocked the analysand because the latter was little and not smart, although he tried to show how he could create something new in computer programs. Mother called the boy "doll" as he had a lovely appearance, and that humiliated him in front of his friends. Patient called his relationships with parents "a full-scale invasion" as he was totally controlled, did not have his room or anything of his own. "I entered the institute, got away from home and got into a company of drug users. There I was accepted the way I was." At the same time, X. met a much older boy who did not let him "get dissolved in drugs. He would invite me home, talk to me for hours quietly, calmly and confidently." At the same time, analysand got invited into a rock band – he played the bass guitar. That was when he changed his name. He has a tattoo of it on his neck, in big letters. Since then, people started to call him, for instance, Guy. He chose the new name spontaneously. "It was like a new me, a different one. I could talk. Before that I would stand aside and be afraid, but then I relaxed for the first time and said: "Hello. I'm Guy."

When I became Guy, everything changed. Mother said she would cut out the skin from my neck, so that she wouldn't see it on the tattoo. "We chose a name for you," father yelled, and I said I was Guy, and I was the one who picked it. When I start doing something new or feel frightened, I become guy, and my behavior changes immediately, as Guy always has to cope with it. My father did not recognize me when I was X., but started to recognize when I became Guy. X. always needed a lot of effort to be seen and appreciated. When I achieved something, I was Guy. And I am tired, I want to be X." "And you need to kill rusnia for that?" "Yes."

What we have today in our practice can be connoted as connection of traumas from non-verbalized actual ones to verbalized repressed ones due to actualization, and it causes the question of separation. According to Freud (1913/2012) symbolic murder of father must be carried out by every son, but it is a complicated process, and X. looked for various ways as Guy. It was important for him to kill the enemy not as Guy, but as X. To pick his weapon. He chose language. As since February 24th he speaks Ukrainian. This case made me think about the way the general influences the subjective and vice versa. Every manifestation of the unconscious is classified as a signifier. Exteriorizations of the unconscious belong to various realities: Gesture, word, action, although among all the realities, it is the speech that gives the most correct manifestation of the order in the unconscious. Nasio (1998), for instance, suggested that dreams were a king's highway to the unconscious for Freud while it the king's highway for Lacan was speech. Lacan therefore introduced the tool to differentiate language and speech activity, termed "Lalangue," to show how the unconscious exists in language. Moreover, due to these manifestations, the analytical theory states that the unconscious is structured like language (Lacan, 1966; Lacan, 1972–1973/2011). This neologism that combines an article and a noun serves to differentiate the language of the unconscious and the language in its linguistic sense. It is the "lalangue" that analysand speaks to express his intersubjective experience. "Lalangue" is the language of sense, full of senses. What does the tattoo on analysand's neck mean – his new name Guy? We may think that the letters include a part of the fracture, and what is written has a similarity to language as structure. And if this word is written on the real body, then it is literally a "lalangue" that the unconscious uses to produce its effects. We give it a sense in accordance to the body we have. Psychoanalysis that uncovers senses is always attentive to the body as it also speaks. Of course, we mean the image of the body. But why not pay attention to the signs written on the body, as they are also addressed to the Other? One cannot access the knowledge without going through the body. Analysand X. would wear "patriotic" hoodies to every session. They had writings: "We don't kill enough rusnia," or "Freedom is our Mother," or "Burn the Kremlin," "Ukrainians are free." When one lacks for words, clothes can also become an act of speech.

Language and speech let one think about the separation way of the subject as well. If a child is like a foreigner at the beginning, as it speaks its own language, with time he or she has to accept the language of the Others. Later, in the process of separation, language can also become an important act to use in other circumstances. We know that there is a signifier when it is attached to a group of signifiers: One of the many. Lacan posed that a signifier is only a signifier for other signifiers. War is a chain of signifiers for every person. It means, when a signifier appears, it calls for other signifiers from the past and foresees the appearance of future signifiers. I do not know what I say – the signifier is addressed to another signifier, that it to the grand Other. Subject does not know what phrase this one is going to be connected with. "I want to kill rusnia" is tightly connected with other signifiers that led to realization of the sense of this connection. What does the subject not know? How the word is going to influence the Other. The symptom as a signifier is a relevant suffering. By relevant, we mean the message that speaks of our past – the one we did not know. The meaning of the symptom as signifier is that it is manifested at a necessary moment as an irreplaceable element that raises a question to analysand and analyst: How is it that everything re-occurs? That means the symptom appears at the necessary moment, and although the subject suffers, it gives a new light to his life. Who could have thought! analysand says, facing the sign, the reason of suffering as a manifestation of the unconscious. Who could have thought that a symptom that made something clear to me appeared at the moment when I could grasp it? And this is the key moment of analysand's discovery.

Lacan (1964/2007) in his seminar *The Four Fundamental Concepts of Psychoanalysis* talks about two fundamental notions – alienation and separation – as those that are greatly significant for psychoanalysis. These are logical operations, and French psychoanalyst reflects upon them through the concept of phantasm. Lacan suggested about alienation and separation not in terms of psychology as separation from mother and parents in general, but his view is much broader. He emphasized about the truth, logic and place. The truth does not want to be articulated, and alienation would raise a question to the subject: it's either this or that, either trick or treat, and if we choose treat, it is not only the treat we lose. How does one live with such important losses? What has value in life then – subject asks. He faces the choice, because it is impossible at the same time – being a Ukrainian and loving, for example, Russia. Feeling Ukrainian and speak Russian, finally be self-reliant and free from instructions of others. He must make a choice, and the subject does it in the act of speech. Like my analysand. "I want to kill rusnia."

Separation lets us choose, separate ourselves from the Other with the help of language and speech, that is castration, as it takes place in the symbolic. There is already the word and the space to articulate the symptoms and then call it with words. As a result of psychoanalytical work, analysand gets the opportunity to choose as well as to wish, which means he can have his borders, estimate the significance of Others, relations with them, and have an ability to bear the traumas of being. The word itself that is the beginning of language and speech today plays an important role for us in seeing ourselves as Ukrainians.

Humboldt (1835/1999), a German philologist, proposed that language is a world that lies between the world of outer events and the inner world of human being. Language forms and sorts thinking, thoughts and actions, intentions and goals, represents one's own Ego and life principles – actually all those things that appear due to separation. The Other that was interested in inhibition of separation used all means from not letting choose to threats and tortures. Language policy is the most powerful technology of influencing nations, and language wars are an inevitable part of information wars. Language is a weapon, and language wars usually go along real wars, but often start before them. We have this experience. Today this theory, together with the theory of nationalism, has become our motto in the war with Russia. From the statement that there is no language to the statement there is no Ukrainian nation. Language has become a geopolitical object. These messages, in my opinion, are tightly connected with stories that each of us goes through in his or her own discourse intersubjectively.

Conclusion

Something must occur between analyst and analysand who freezes due to endless repetition of actual trauma. It is something that we can think of as a linguistic dimension of war in the logic of contribution to trans-subjective manifestations of separation from defining the personal to the common in the act of speech and subjective ways of overcoming traumas. Because following Freud, we have to accept the tragic severity of human condition. Certainly, sometimes we are desperate – it is the tragic fate of psychoanalysis and psychoanalysts. However, here in Ukraine we know that when cannons speak, psychoanalysis exists, as it gives the subject an opportunity to express themselves even when there are no words. When a trauma that cannot be articulated goes all the way from total silence and numbness to almost primal cry that is bound to death, to whining and wailing, and then later to words – articulation does take place in psychoanalytical framework. As trauma must go through verbal realization. The goal of the psychoanalyst in this case is to help the patient make up his mind to go along the way of processing the mental experience in speech and connecting to the symbolic order, in which the non-verbalized Real can have speech realization of the Symbolic and become clear in the Imaginary. The goal of psychoanalysis then is to restore the lost spaces, or precisely their meanings, finding a different form of expression to the unarticulated reality.

References

Barthelemy, G. (1997). Fromentin et l'écriture du désert. Fromentin et l'écriture du désert. L'harmattan.

Corbin, A. (2018). *A history of silence: From the renaissance to the present day*. John Wiley & Sons.

Dolar, M. (2006). *A voice and nothing more*. MIT Press.

Ferrell, R. (2006). *Passion in theory: Conceptions of Freud and Lacan*. Routledge.

Freud, S. (1899/2022). *The interpretation of dreams*. DigiCat.

Freud, S. (1905). Three essays on the theory of sexuality. *Standard Edition*, Vol. 7, 125–243.

Freud, S. (1913/2012). *Totem and taboo*. Routledge.

Freud, S. (1919/2017). The uncanny. In *Romantic writings* (pp. 318–325). Routledge.

Freud, S. (1920/2015). Beyond the pleasure principle. *Psychoanalysis and History*, 17(2), 151–204.

Freud, S. (1937/1959). Analysis terminable and interminable. In *Collected papers* (Vol. 5, pp. 316–357). Basic Books.

Klein, M. (1987). *Selected Melanie Klein*. Simon and Schuster.

Lacan, J. *Les formations de l'inconscient. Séminaire 1957–1958*. A.L.I.

Lacan, J. (1957). La relation d'objet et les structures freudiennes. *Bulletin de psychologie*, 10(7), 426–430.

Lacan, J. (1968). *The language of the self: The function of language in psychoanalysis*. JHU Press.

Lippi, S. (2014). La voix sur le divan. Musique sacrée, opéra, techno: Jean-Michel Vives, Aubier, 2012. Cahiers de psychologie clinique, 2, 239–242.

Loraux, N. (2002). *The mourning voice: An essay on Greek tragedy*. Cornell University Press.

Mallarmé, S. (2011). Collected poems: A bilingual edition. University of California Press.

Medvedieva, O. (2024). How long is forever?' 'Sometimes only one second'": The measurement of time as a factor of the unconscious and features of its transformation in the subject's traumatic experience. *Ukrainian Psychoanalytic Journal*, 2(1), 32–44. https://doi.org/10.32782/upj/2024-1-5

Nasio, J. D. (1998). *Five lessons on the psychoanalytic theory of Jacques Lacan*. SUNY Press.

Segal, H. (2006). *Dream, phantasy and art*. Routledge.

Vivès, J. M. (2013). The voice in psychoanalysis. *Reverso*, 35(66), 19–24.

Von Humboldt, W. (1835/1999). *Humboldt: 'On language': On the diversity of human language construction and its influence on the mental development of the human species*. Cambridge University Press.

Chapter 5

The Mental Void

Impact of War on Non-Neurotic Structures

Olga Pavlovska and Nina Kokoilo

War is a real paroxysm in the existence of modern societies.
Roger Caillois, "Man and the Sacred"

The war impacts the human subject on both the intersubjective and intrapsychic levels. The experience of war makes psychoanalysts, and their analysands face numerous questions on various levels. Understanding the impact of ongoing war requires attention to the processes of constructing subjectivity and symbolization of mental experience. In our view, the analytic creation of representations related to drives and objects of satisfaction serves toward digesting personal experiences (including those of wars), which defines subjectivization (Pavlovska, 2023).

We define the process of subjectivization as the formation of a subject in relationship with the Other through their intersubjective connection. This relationship is always paradoxical. The formation of a basis for satisfaction of the subject's wishes depends on the position of the Other within the subject's psyche. The creative process of designing a connection with the Other was described by Freud, Winnicott, Lacan, Green, and other psychoanalytic scholars. Observations of life and psychoanalytical practice confirm that the process of building human subjectivity involves a series of identifications, such as attempting to become similar to the Other by obeying the Other's desires for us. On the other hand, individuals can refuse to obey, seeking to separate, which activates aggression (Lesourd, 2011). Such processes in the development of subjectivity acknowledge the role of the subject's drives and the Other's response to them. Moreover, the consequences of the subject's drives when meeting the Other become manifested in the activity of the Ego subject. In this formulation, the Other is differentiated from the figures of concrete "other" in the psyche, such as the primary figure of a

DOI: 10.4324/9781032660257-6

"good enough mother" (Winnicott, 2016), who provides care to the child, allowing the presence of helplessness of a child who is not yet capable to satisfy the drives (Winnicott, 1980). Green (1999a) termed the primary figure of the Other "a similar other." In turn, Lacan (1958) defined it as a "little other," emphasizing various psychic possibilities for the Other's internal representation. Shared in these theories is the view that human subjectivity is built through the relation with the Other, and human being can only organize themselves and their desires through the Other, both the similar and the dissimilar Other (Green, 2000).

The psychoanalyst's attention on the intrapsychic level is typically focused on the sources of the patient's mental life, such as the drives or psychosexuality, viewed as forms of primary mental activity. Certainly, the intrapsychic is viewed as marked by human dependence on biological functions. Thus, the intersubjective and intrapsychic levels always exist in the mutual intersection: in the process of analyzing a patient's subjectivity, many psychoanalysts seek to pay attention to both the inversions of the subject's drives and the desires for connection with the Other, which often form acceptance or refusal to submit. Thus, human function heavily depends on the presence and role of the internalized Other. The Other serves as the point of construction and deconstruction of human subjectivity. The Other within the subject's psyche (i.e., the representation of Other) can be signified as a persecutor, the judge of desires, or a deadly authority that destroys the manifestations of life and creativity (Green, 1975, 1998, 1999a, 2000, 2001).

This understanding of subjectivity makes the subject-object bond and separation between them more complicated because it does not reduce the object representation to the image of a real object while emphasizing that the object's response is related to the subject's drives. In human reality, the imperfections of an object's responses to the subject's drives are common, and many individuals cannot integrate their drives together with their Ego functioning, thus creating breaks or voids in the capacity to experience integration (Green, 1999a; Lutenberg, 2007). Therefore, every mental structure, including in Oedipal neuroses, is viewed as marked traumatic experiences that are not integrated into the psyche while remaining influential in the mental lives of most individuals. However, these challenges are especially significant in the mental structures of individuals with non-neurotic personalities, for whom the traumatic experiences with the Other and the breaks from reality are more profound. Green (1999a, 2000a, 2001) was among psychoanalytic scholars who suggested the vicissitude of mental life among individuals with such non-neurotic structures.

In contrast to non-neurotic patients, working with the neurotic subject offers an opportunity for the psychoanalyst to follow their patient's mental activity, whether drive-based or related to fantasy, which is typically organized around denial and repression in mental functioning. On the other hand, the mental functioning of non-neurotic subjects is predominated by more disorganizing defense mechanisms such as repression, splitting, or negative hallucinations, which resemble thinking disorders. Psychoanalysts who work with such non-neurotic analysands often stress the importance of the patient's increased capability to create representations and use them, including as mechanisms against depression, which can limit affective responses in general (Pavlovska, 2023).

Thereby, non-neurotic structures are believed to be formed around the unconscious psyche that is mostly characterized by a lack of organization. We have observed that if these patients face destructive forces, whether inner or outer, their formed structure is easily damaged, which then results in either addiction, melancholy, or acting out. These defensive reactions appear as "organized disorganization" (e.g., the organization of self as contained by relation with an addictive object). Their defensive maneuvers against excessive excitation are often aimed at protecting mental activity from being seized by destructive processes. Considering these theoretical and clinical observations, we, as Ukrainian psychoanalysts, have been faced with new challenges of understanding mental processes and clinical engagement with non-neurotic patients under conditions of ongoing full-scale war.

Wars force all human beings affected by them to face a traumatic environment. Indeed, human interaction with various acts of war (e.g., bombings) and their real losses while also facing the terrifying images of murdered people and ruined houses actualizes the archaic layers of what we understand as mental representations. The Other takes up the position of a tyrant totalitarian object who forces the subject to face mental helplessness. Doubtless, being a victim of war is traumatic for all human psyches, including not just in an external threat to life but in the excessive inner aggression (rage) joined together with a lack of external aggression, which can result in a sense of passivity and powerlessness. War becomes a forced disruption that, among other forms of violence, also interrupts normal human preoccupations with relationships, work, home, habits, and pleasure or, in short, everything that defines most human values. War becomes an experience of extreme collective disturbance as human beings face catastrophic experiences and terrors.

Notably, one of the most significant aspects of psychic function among non-neurotic patients, even outside of such conditions as wars, is their preoccupation with a sense of inner void, which marks these patients' inability to represent or symbolize their experiences. Typically their mental strategies are focused on avoiding all forms of suffering (Lutenberg, 2007). For many of them, to accept the experiences of suffering is internally interpreted as a type of destruction (Green, 2000a). They tend to believe that their suffering will last forever, destroying any capabilities of their psyche to gain satisfying experience or form expectations for the future. Such a vortex of emptiness and hopelessness is typically described by non-neurotic patients as endless suffering. Thus, in this chapter, we expound on this notion while also illustrating how non-neurotic patients pursue addictive objects in order to negate or escape their suffering. On the other hand, as we highlight, when they also face a catastrophe like war, the external reality can provide an opportunity, usually unavailable in "normal times," to materialize their terrors in reality. This war intrusion can serve to reveal the empty void of their non-represented experience and help them recognize its presence in their internal mental space.

On the Experiences of the Void

Psychoanalytic theorists, grounded in various psychoanalytical traditions, suggest that in the contemporary world, the experience of an empty void or the absent and negative tends to define many clinical cases. In psychoanalytic scholarship, this void has been described by many (Bollas, 2017; Botella & Botella, 2005; Green, 1999a; Kohon, 1999; Lutenberg, 2007; McDougall, 1992; Perelberg, 2017; Rosas, 2023). For instance, Lutenberg introduced the term "structural void," specifying that, from a metaphysical point of view, this void appears when the human psyche experiences a hiatus between its symbiotic psychic vector and the narcissistic structure. Thus, the "structural mental void" is viewed as a primary basic configuration of the psyche that coexists along with the accompanying and compensating sub-structures such as the psychotic, phobic, hysterical, and so forth. The clinical phenomenon of "mental void" is seen as manifested in associative process disorders, which can be experienced during sessions (e.g., excessive silence or reactions not marked by identifiable repression).

In addition, analysts recognize these processes in severe negative therapeutic reactions or massive regression.

Green (1986b) offered several conceptual models of this phenomenon, referring to them as the "white series," "white" psychosis, "white" mourning, "white" anxiety, and the negative hallucination. He described states of the psyche in which the subject is able to develop the capacity to stand against the chaos of drives and psychotic anxieties. "White" psychosis, he noted, is the psychosis without the presence of delusion because it "attacks the thought itself,' not letting thinking fill in the void because it lacks reasoning (Green, 1986b). Green emphasized that this hiatus in thinking among non-neurotic analysands is extremely common. Their psychic void serves to disorganize the psyche, filling it with delusion, addictive objects, or perverse thinking. Moreover, Green drew attention to the processes of erasing common in such psychic functions, which is not related to neurotic normal repression. As a result of this activity, non-neurotic patients form a "hole" in their psyche that sucks in their mental meanings and thoughts, especially meanings and thoughts related to the central purpose or reason for the existence of this "hole" (Green, 1998).

Within intersubjective cultural dimensions of the contemporary world, the phenomenon of void is found in rigid ideologies, in cultures of omnipotence and reductionism. The crisis of desire in cases of such void-making is solved through the formation of a powerful demand for the Other, who is sought out to fill in the lack at all costs. These "white" subjects resist complicated thinking, reject attachment, and fundamentally refuse to invest their libido into objects. Green stressed that their mental functioning is typically based on a pseudo-structure which covers empty voids in subject's Ego. These pseudo-structures can only experience their links with the Other as being limited by their similarities with the Other, rejecting all forms of otherness as a threat (Rosas, 2023).

The psyche of non-neurotic patients is disturbed by all processes perceived as devastation, certainly including the devastation of war. The mere absence of objects signifies for them the presence of void and death (Winnicott, 1991). Trauma is experienced not just connected to the identifiable event but because it was expected (i.e., but not occurred). The tyranny of its absence imbues it with lasting power. The failure of responses from the environment to the subject's needs is one key aspect of this trauma. The catastrophe of devastation also makes the subject lose hope, not trusting the other while attempting to defend against betrayal and pain (Escande, 2016).

Unmet expectation create a mental economy without a future, while overly anxious emotional experiences that subjects cannot bear forecloses their capacity to mentalize and properly somaticize (e.g., in writings of Marty, M'Uzan, McDougall). The typical appearance of addiction and melancholy marks such experiences (Escande, 2016). The following clinical illustrations discuss further these aspects of non-neurotic experiences of the void and the impact of war on these experiences. The case of J (Pavlovska) and the case of K (Kokoilo) are presented below.

Case of J

Before the War

In our early sessions together, J explained that when he was 16, he decided to formally adopt a brand new name with a reference to an ancient war leader, legally changing his simple birth name on all of his documents. When treatment commenced, J was 22 years old. He entered treatment with complaints about what he described as a "strange and exhausting" relationship with a girlfriend. He discussed his dislike of her "dependence" on him and often shared his wishes to "get rid" of what he experiences as a "torturing relationship." What I (Pavlovska) gathered in our sessions was different: their relationship was merely a correspondence with view occasional meetings because the young woman lived in a different city. They had no sexual relationship, which also seemed to bother J. J's reactions appeared to be focused on his interpretations of their correspondence: the young woman would often not respond to his messages for days at a time, after which she would re-appear online, continuing their" relationship." J's reactions to her "disappearing" and the fact he did not understand its reasons or discuss this with her resulted in significant outbursts of rage and desperation. In a fit of rage, he described deleting his social media accounts or blocking her. In his rage, he described episodes of bursting out in tears or throwing his electronic devices against the wall. Only some time into our treatment, J shared that he worked in the IT sphere, and I learned that his entire relational and work life, more or less, has taken place in the virtual world since he was 10 years old. J described himself as a professional gamer who worked in game development, including participating in professional online championships. Failures in gaming or in his communication with other players always also caused J fits of rage, growing his "cemetery" of electronic devices thrown against the wall.

His relationships with colleagues followed a similar scenario. J reported finding a job, which at first inspired him with new possibilities and expectations. Several months into his work, he described experiences of not understanding what his bosses or colleagues "wanted from him." After work meetings, which he said he could not decipher, he would get angry, including repeatedly telling himself that he was "dumb." It became clear that he lacked the capacity to read or relate to others. Within a few months of each new job, J described becoming desperate and feeling exhausted. His tasks would take him more and more time, he would get distracted from work, and eventually become physically sick. In our analysis, J often complained about his "bad health." According to him, he "suffered" from numerous "allergies." J reported that he was diagnosed with asthma in his childhood but indicated that by his early adulthood, he no longer experienced any asthma attacks.

J also reported that he continually moved homes (i.e., every six months or within one year) and that he changed jobs and cities with similar frequency. At the time of our analysis, J ended up spending most of his time in a single city, where we worked together in analysis for four years. His social connections remained limited to occasional in-person meetings with several acquaintances.

Family History

J's parents were married young when they were only 18 years old because of the pregnancy with J. When J was 2, his parents divorced. His early memories include remembering scenes of parental conflicts and his fruitless attempts to attract attention to himself in order to distract parents from fighting. After the divorce, J went to live with his mother and her parents. J described his mother as being utterly dependent on her mother (J's maternal grandmother). His mother also was married several more times. J described that neither feelings nor wishes or thoughts were ever openly shared in his family but that the most common pattern of relating was manipulation. J recalled his growing up as lacking any warmth or connection. Both his mother and his grandmother would routinely "forget" J's asthma or allergies, and his own view seemed to be that he was "not important" to anyone in his family.

J's father was predominantly absent. Until J was a teen, he recalled having no calls or communication from his father, but then when he became a teen, his father suddenly began calling him frequently to complain about his business failures while calling J "darling." In our work, it became clear that J's father remained connected to J predominately through requests for money and loans but seemed to lack any interest in J's life.

During our work, J appeared to become calmer and began to relate his fits of rage with the feelings of a profound flooding sense of absence related to his perception of lack in their response to him. It became clear that the result of persistent failures of the holding environment (Winnicott, 1991) resulted in a lack of development and weakness of his mental structures. The question of his own place in relationships with others seemed paramount to J. He could identify that his persistent search for new homes replaced his struggle to relate. J's internal representations could not be sustained and were easily erased, while his psychic excitations could flood his Ego and distract him from the relationally empty void. His addiction to gaming became one of the main organizing psychic defenses.

The War

For J, as for millions of Ukrainians, the Russian war against Ukraine started in 2014. At the time, he lived with his family in the East of Ukraine, and he directly witnessed the realities of the Russian military invasion and ensuing chaos. J could identify that it was at that moment in time when his family completely fell apart. His grandmothers, mother, and aunt all fled to different countries in Europe. J and his father stayed in Ukraine, relocating to other cities. It became impossible for J (or his family) to come back home. Notably, it was then that J changed his name to one of an ancient war leader.

Strikingly, J seemed unable to discuss the loss of his home to war never. When asked, J responded with rationalizations that stressed that leaving his birth city was his "choice" and that he was planning to move "anyway" in order to "study." Losing his home to war marked his perpetual search for new places to live.

J faced the full-scale Russian invasion while he lived in Kyiv. Unlike most Ukrainians, who seemed to share severe anxiety while awaiting the invasion for several months in the winter of 2022, J seemed unaffected. He reported life as usual, gaming for hours, obsessively studying cryptocurrency, and describing being "mesmerized" for hours by varied economic charts.

When the invasion began, I (Pavlovska) moved out of Kyiv for safety, although our work was interrupted only for several days. Almost all my analysands either fled the city or joined the army in those early days of full-scale war. I observed that J remained frozen in his actions. He appeared to say nothing about our shared outer reality as if it did not exist, and during our sessions, he went on discussing his work stubbornly. After several weeks of this pattern, I asked him directly about his experience of war. J appeared not to know what to say and appeared unable to even think about it. Once, late in the evening, he called me and shared that he was terrified because his friend acted "very strangely and aggressively." In speaking with J, I realized that his friend was having a psychotic break caused by fear of shelling. I explained to J what was happening and talked him through what he should do. After his event, we began discussing little by little about J's experiences of war. Certainly, his primary complaints remained mostly focused on his physical condition. J reported that his allergies returned and talked about having a difficult time "breathing through the nose." J shared that he could not sleep and that, from time to time, he wanted to just quit analysis and leave. His anxiety would then take hold of him as he discussed that country borders were closed for men because of military conditions.

In my observations, I could see that his physical challenges represented feelings of varied intrusions of not only varied (unresponded to) illnesses in his childhood but also experiences of intrusion from outer reality, past and present. Notably, my interpretation was not based on my analytic reflection but on direct living reaction to common traumatic reality for us as a psychoanalyst and an analysand. To emphasize, the profound influence and the intrusion of war into the space where intrapsychic and intersubjective intersected, an attack on our joint mental container held by me as a psychoanalyst and J as an analysand, which helped be both connected and separate.

Shared experience of this aggressive intrusion into our reality lets us find and materialize the figure of the Other, which, prior to this moment, would typically slip away from symbolization. It became obvious that the Other for J was the attacker on the mental surface of his transitional space (i.e., using Winnicott's idea of transitional space from bodily reality to outer reality). The void and absence of mental representations revealed the status of the Other in his psyche from his childhood: the absent Other who caused J pain and rage. The existence of the actual outer aggressor in the Russian military and Russian government let us symbolize another important aspect of the Other in his psyche: the Other as a persecutor who does not want to satisfy his wishes or to live but who made J feel doomed and vengeful at the same time.

For a long time, it seemed that J could not hold me as a separate person in his mind or be interested in anything about me outside our analytic hour.

In my counter-transference, I fantasized about provoking him with stories about myself and my reality. I began to imagine that I could tell him about my experience working as a translator in a military project and that hearing it, he would come awake and be able to talk about hard feelings connected with war. This fantasy let me realize the importance of non-intrusion into his mental reality of his inner Other until J himself could become ready.

Instead, J began to discuss termination. We agreed on a date for several months out. J shared that he imagined that our final session would fall on a Monday, but he stressed that he was the one to decide which Monday, only a week prior to our last meeting. It was important for him to make this choice, and I agreed.

During those several months, J appeared more calm and kinder, including in his curiosity toward me. He began to ask whether I had children and then asked if I could share their names. He stated that he "adored" the name of my daughter. He even brought a dream to our last session:

> *I walk not far away from my home, circling around the neighborhood, and suddenly I realize there are bears and that I should go back home immediately. As I move around in a circle to avoid the bears, the distance to home is the same if I go forward or backward. It's just a matter of choice.*

At another point, J smiled when looking at me when he shared: "You know, I had a virtual friend in a game, and she had the same name as you. She'd always fly to me [in the game she was a bird] and explain how to advance to a new level."

Concluding Comment

After J left treatment, I felt anxious about his capacity to transform his experience into words because of his tendency toward somatization. I felt we did not have enough time to process his experiences or to work with his defensive structures. On the other hand, I believe that J's decision on the structure and timing of how to end our analysis provided him with a new position toward the Other. Possibly for the first time with another human being, he could be the master of the situation. Because of the therapeutic space we created and his new self-perception, J chose to risk losing an object without risking losing himself at the same time. For me, J's case became an illustration of the process described by Freud about a child's play with a reel. J became capable of playing with self-representation and accomplishing some integration. The final part of our analysis mostly represented this kind of play under my "supervision" as a psychoanalyst. What emerged between us could not be expressed in words before then. As Green (1999a) noted, mental activity at the beginning of life is typically organized in the hallucinatory register seeking the return of experiences of satisfaction – and the first stage of the anti-depressive process. The second stage, he stressed, included the creation of representations of the object. Then the mental process that allows the person to deal with loss can commence (Green, 1999a). J's work, including his termination, as well as our shared intersubjective experiences of war, became another step toward J's capacity to face his losses and his affective responses.

Case of K

At the time of initiating treatment with me (Kokoilo), the analysand, a woman, was 35 years old and married. She sought out help two months after the full-scale Russian military invasion of Ukraine. During the most dangerous and anxious weeks of the war, as Russia attacked Kyiv and the surrounding areas, she remained in the city with her family. K reported that her mental state deteriorated abruptly at that time as Russian rockets and bombs hit the city, air raid sirens blared, and terrible news caused her panic attacks and obsessive thoughts. She described that her extreme early agitation then turned into apathy and hopelessness. She stated that on most days, she could not eat, did not change her clothes and that she forced herself out of the state of shock to care for her young child. After several months, she evacuated with her child and her mother to Germany. Once a refugee, she described developing severe depression and reported feelings of constant guilt and the sensation of "being lost." In addition, K reported symptoms of bulimia.

Personal History

K indicated that she was "the first unwanted child" of her mother. Mother told her that she became pregnant with K by "accident" and then made several attempts to end the pregnancy but that K's father "prevented abortion" and instead offered K's mother marriage. During her growing up, K often heard her father complain of "sacrificing" himself for K and "suffering" because of his decision, which left K feeling confused and guilty. K's mother, from her memories, was cold, cruel, and endlessly criticizing, whose typical reaction to conflict was to withdraw her affection, including not speaking with K or her siblings for months at a time. When K became a mother herself, she acknowledged to herself for the first time that her family lacked love or affection. K then turned toward her own child as her "whole world."

During our analysis, K repeatedly recalls several childhood experiences. In one of them, when K was about five years old, she was left alone with her three-year-old brother for several hours. She and her brother played with matches left lying around and started a fire. They were saved and uninjured, but the parents' response was to punish K as the older child. Their punishment included burning K's fingers with a lighter to "teach a lesson" that fire was dangerous. In another recollection, when K was 13, she recalled her father began beating her. K recalled that at the time, her father lost his job and began drinking heavily. K's memories of the beatings included scenes of being punched in the stomach, her face, and her head until K collapsed. She described those moments as feeling utterly helpless, shocked, and numb, which she mentioned were her only way of not feeling physical pain. In K's memories, her mother is around the house but would never interfere in the abuse. Moreover, in those years, K was described as either being the one to comfort her mother when her mother was distressed or being faced with her mother's months-long silent treatment. In her teen years, K developed bulimia. She also entered into a romantic relationship with a drug addict who overdosed and died, which led K to develop severe symptoms of depression that required hospitalization.

K reported that after several abusive relationships, she "finally" found a partner whom she trusted and liked and whom she found emotionally available. She distanced herself from her family of origin. She became pregnant and excitedly turned her life toward motherhood. While she shared that she "always expected a catastrophe to strike," until the invasion she felt she was able to live life more as she hoped. The invasion, her forced migration, and her refugee status forced her to live with her mother again, who engaged in treating K with the same disdain and silent treatment. For K, her very psychic survival began to hinge on her returning back to Ukraine.

Treatment

The catastrophe of war for K, who has been running away from her trauma, resulted in facing the invasion with non-integrated or weakly integrated non-neurotic psychic structures. The invasion and its impact were abrupt and profoundly violent. This event impeded K's capacity to cope, paralyzing her. Violence and terror of war resonated with her personal history (e.g., beatings and fire were common in Russian attacks on Ukrainian civilians).

Reactions from her childhood to unbearable suffering emerged at this time as well. Just as in her early years, K reacted by blocking her experience with distancing reactions, such as describing her beatings as "not so bad." In response to her words at one of the sessions, we had the following dialogue:

Psychoanalyst: "If you let yourself experience the terror or what happens to you, you wouldn't survive, so the only solution for you is freezing and being alone in that terror."

K: "You know, I once complained to a colleague about not knowing what to do about an abusive boss in my office, and she said there was always a way out of any situation. I was so disappointed by what she said; what could she possibly know? I think that looking for a way out is just prolonging hopelessness and pain."

This exchange is typical, illustrating K's defense against being flooded by affect. Searching for solutions causes a state of mental pain, which leads to growing hopelessness. Mental emptiness then appears to be the result of dissociation, serving a protective function, which pushes against the limits of the ability to bear mental struggle, especially when facing the catastrophe alone. In the course of our psychoanalytical work, K continually faced her non-symbolized terror.

During our work, an earthquake occurred in Turkey. During one of the sessions, K shared that she numbly watched all available videos from the events, looking for shots of people buried under collapsed houses. She stated that she was afraid of seeing any such images in Ukraine. She noted that she could not emotionally bear it. Notably, the event that really shook her and made her face her terror was being stuck in a car wash facility, which devastated and awakened her from a state of numbness. This experience at the car wash became an opening for having more affective reactions to memories of what happened to her during childhood. The event left me encountering both the integrated and non-integrated experiences of trauma. The emotion of helplessness links the scenes of K's past and present: being severely beaten, facing the violence of the Russian invasion, and her mother's neglect.

Conclusion

In work with non-neurotic patients, the catastrophe, such as the war, reflects the catastrophes that already happened to these individuals. In analytic work during the war, the possibility is not only in the integration of the traumatic reality itself but also in acknowledgment of other traumas, often unformulated and unintegrated, along with the failures of expectations of what the patient needed from the Other. These relational failures compromised such patients' lifelong and basic feelings of safety and their capacity for mental continuity. These failures of holding result in their continued fears of falling apart because of the lack of object representation in their psyche. The source of damage to their mental structures is typically an event that has not been mentalized or processed, which prevents mourning, including mourning of betrayed relational expectations. These challenges form the basis of how non-neurotically organized individuals face profoundly destructive external realities such as the war.

Certainly, in our cases, we highlighted the possibilities for psychic repair. However, like all clinicians who work with non-neurotic analysands, we recognize that such patients face many regressive movements. Recurring realities that repeat prior childhood scenes that caused severe anxiety or pain can contribute to regressive defenses of intellectualization, repetition compulsion, or derealization. Moreover, if the Other experienced by such patients as possessing a narcissistic capacity to control or destroy, which the patient is powerless to affect, both the patient and any internal representations can remain in their internal void (Botella & Botella, 2005). The lost fragments of the Ego in the patient's psyche give no space for desire, libido, or subjectivity. Notably, many non-neurotic analysands create traps (mental and relational) in the process of constructing their internal and external subjectivity.

A human being is always in the process of constructing a self. Human subjectivity is based on the capacity to hold, create, and reformat new experiences during the entire lifespan. At times, human beings have to fix or glue together their worlds from pieces left in the wake of a catastrophic reality, which at times is literally the Ukrainian experience under the conditions of war. During the war, the psychoanalyst's own mental reality is involved not only in the analytical process but is also affected by the experiences of war and its collective charge. All Ukrainians today live in a space of collective trauma that, for many, also resonates with multiple traumas stemming from their past. Many of these traumas are generational: Ukraine has been the land that historian Timothy Snyder (2015) referred to as the "bloodlands": the land that faced wars, genocides, resettlements, deportations, forced hunger, and protracted periods of control by totalitarian regimes. Nearly every Ukrainian family has "unburied" trauma in their history.

As psychoanalysts, we recognize that war always causes massive subjective and collective regression. Traumas of various natures and magnitudes are re-activated by war all the time. In terms of war, individuals exist on the edge of their capabilities to symbolize what happens. Life amidst the real war, as well as the virtual war online, further complicates the relationship of safety and victimhood, often openly shared with and between the psychoanalyst and the analysands.

Impediments and anxieties of non-neurotic patients can prevent them from creating the mental connections needed to understand and face their reality, such as historicizing life events and methods of responding to them. Non-integrated psychic states also require help toward integration from the Other (i.e., the psychoanalyst). Importantly, if the traumatic experience is perceived as having returned, in part or fully, and is brought into the transference field, a person might have a chance to work toward integration. Trauma, which was previously seen only as a shadow in personal history, is given a shape, and the created representation, which becomes a memory, can fill in the mental gaps, not letting a person slip into the void. Psychoanalyst in conditions of war requires dynamic creative capacity to contain in order to create reflexive shared movement with analysand in order to support their symbolic meaning-making. Changes in psychoanalytic work due to the war encouraged Ukrainian psychoanalysts to deal with new observations and reflect on them (e.g., Lagutin, 2023; Pustovoyt, 2023; Velykodna, 2023; Zaleskyi, 2023).

Following the ideas of post-Lacanian scholars such as Brune et al. (2019), we also view this task as the creation of the mediation object. A mediation object is an object that can support a symbolization process, bringing it forth from the unrepresented sensory motor perceptions toward primary and secondary symbolization processes (see Khrystenko in Velykodna et al., 2023). This approach may aid the development of mental space in which the non-symbolized and unthinkable experience acquires forms. This process has also been referred to by Botella and Botella (2005) as "the work of figurability," focusing on the expression through words and speech. Not only can this process fill in the specific mental lacunae of the analysand within the psychic void, but it helps them recover the flow of drives and their neurotic function.

War in Ukraine continues. We wish to end with the acknowledgment that it is challenging to understand the processes while being inside their "fire." War is an invasive experience, literally and psychically, and is always experienced as violence. In Ukraine today, we are attempting to create the "framing structure" (Green, 1999a) for our analysands as well as to learn to theorize about pain and complex feelings without only speaking of the implicit. We are simultaneously searching for the missing links between the events, images, and symbolic meanings of reality that are ongoing.

References

Bollas, C (2017). *The Shadow of the Object Psychoanalysis of the Unthought Known*. Routledge.

Botella, C., & Botella, S. (2005). *The Work of Psychic Figurability: Mental States without Representation (The New Library of Psychoanalysis)*. Routledge.

Brun, A., Roussillon, R., & Chouvier, B. (2019). *Manuel des médiations thérapeutiques*. Dunod.

Escande, C. (2016). Nostalgia for the future "faces of devastation." *Psychoanalysis Chronicle*, 1(19), 3–10.

Green, A. (1975). The analyst, symbolization and absence in the analytic setting. *International Journal of Psychoanalysis*, 56(1), 1–22.

Green, A. (1986b). *On Private Madness*. Hogarth; International Universities Press.

Green, A. (1998). The primordial mind and the work of the negative. *The International Journal of Psychoanalysis*, 79(4), 649–665.

Green, A. (1999a). *The Work of the Negative*. Free Association Books.

Green, A. (2000). The intrapsychic and intersubjective in psychoanalysis. *The Psychoanalytic Quarterly*, 69(1), 1–39.

Green, A. (2000a). The central phobic position: A new formulation of the free association method. *International Journal of Psychoanalysis*, 81, 429–451.

Green, A. (2001). *Life Narcissism Death Narcissism*. Free Association Books.

Kohon, G. (1999). *The Dead Mother. The work of André Green*. Routledge.

Lacan J. (1958). Les formations de l'inconscient. *Bulletin de psychologie*. 2011/6 (Numéro 516), 519–539.

Lagutin, V. (2023). Psychoanalysis "traumatized" by war. Four clinical illustrations of the vulnerability of the setting. *Ukrainian Psychoanalytic Journal*, 1(3), 18–23. https://doi.org/10.32782/upj/2023-3-3

Lesourd, S. (2011). Primary masochism and subjectivity. *Psychoanalysis Chronicle*, 1(15), 11–20.

Lutenberg, J. M. (2007). Mental void and the borderline patient. In *Resonance of Suffering: Counter in Non-Neurotic Structures*. Karnac.

McDougall J. (1992). The anti-analysand in analysis. In *Plea for a Measure of Abnormality*. Routledge.

Pavlovska, O. (2023). Psychoanalytic work with losses during the war: The Ukrainian experience. *Psychoanalytic Psychology*, 40(4). https://doi.org/10.1037/pap0000479

Perelberg, R.J. (2017). Love and melancholia in the analysis of women by women. *The International Journal of Psychoanalysis*, 98(6). https://doi.org/10.1111/1745-8315.12686

Pustovoyt, M. (2023). Interpreting crisis while in crisis (reflections on psychoanalytic work in hybrid warfare). *Ukrainian Psychoanalytic Journal*, 1(1), 21–26. https://doi.org/10.32782/upj/2023-1-4

Rosas, R.V. (2023). A phantasm called void. *Psychoanalysis Today*. Issue 1. Ghosts. https://www.psychoanalysis.today/en-GB/PT-Articles/Velasco-Rosas153239/Un-fantasma-llamado-vacio.aspx

Snyder T. (2015). *Bloodlands: Europe between Hitler and Stalin*. Vintage.

Velykodna, M. (2023). A Psychoanalyst's experience of working in wartime: On choosing between bad options. *Psychoanalytic Psychology*, 40(4). https://doi.org/10.1037/pap0000480

Velykodna, M., Nalyvaiko, N., Pavlovska, O., Arshevska-Guérin, O., & Butsykin, Y. (2023). Ethical challenges in psychoanalytic practice in wartime: Conference report, Kyiv, Ukraine, 2023, *Psychodynamic Practice*. https://doi.org/10.1080/14753634.2023.2258036

Winnicott, D. W. (1980). Fear of breakdown. *The International Journal of Psychoanalysis*, 61, 351.

Winnicott, D. W. (1991). *Playing and Reality*. Psychology Press.

Winnicott, D. W. (2016). *The collected works of DW Winnicott* (Vol. 12). Oxford University Press.

Zaleskyi, D. (2023). The war of symbols. Symbolization and identity in the context of Russia's war against Ukraine: Analytical view. *Ukrainian Psychoanalytic Journal*, 1(3), 30–34. https://doi.org/10.32782/upj/2023-3-5

Chapter 6

Psychoanalytic Practice in Wartime Ukraine

Challenges to the Ethics

Oksana Arshevska-Guérin, Natalia Nalyvaiko, and Mariana Velykodna

The psychodynamic approach, in its broad meaning, considers ethics an integral dimension of psychoanalytic thinking and practice (Benvenuto, 2018; McWilliams, 2020). Ethics provides analytic practitioners not only with rules that prohibit potentially abusive actions toward the patient (Merlino, 2006) but also with margins of elastic boundaries within which the space of a productive alliance of two subjectivities can unfold (Goodman & Severson, 2016). Moreover, the elaboration of ethical issues in psychoanalysis influenced both psychoanalytic theorizing, emphasizing the role of respect for the subject's truth (Rajchman, 2013) and ethics as a philosophical discipline (Harcourt, 2015).

Current ethical principles and ethical codes of psychoanalytic communities were formulated in historical progress, clarified in response to violations (Burka et al., 2019), and adjusted to the changed external realities, such as the COVID-19 pandemic (Crastnopol, 2021). However, due to the long-term ban of psychoanalysis in the Soviet Union (Butsykin, 2023; Nalyvaiko, 2023c; Velykodna, 2024), independent-Ukraine psychoanalytic societies primarily copied and utilized the ethical codes of their internationally affiliated associations as sufficient for the first sight (Velykodna et al., 2023b).

The sequent Russian invasions of Ukraine in 2014 and 2022 forced Ukrainian psychodynamic specialists to face new challenges in their lives and ability to maintain their practice, posing a threat to thinking and acting under the demands of "ordinary ethics" (Dorozhkin, 2023; Kechur & Haber, 2023; Lagutin, 2023; Lazos, 2023; Pustovoyt, 2023; Velykodna, 2024). Psychoanalysts, as well as other mental health professionals, reported various difficulties in their efforts to deal with these challenges using the existing ethical principles (Filts, 2023; Kechur, 2024; Nalyvaiko, 2023a; Palii, 2023; Romanov, 2023a; Rudenko, 2023), in part due to the

DOI: 10.4324/9781032660257-7

impossibility to maintain the familiar setting and psychoanalytic space with its common time and boundaries (Lagutin, 2023; Nalyvaiko, 2023a).

Since Russia's full-scale war against Ukraine started in 2022, a range of national and international events have been organized to discuss these difficulties. For instance, the series of open meetings of friends of the Ukrainian Psychoanalytic Society (since April 2022), the conference of the Psychoanalytic Psychology and Psychotherapy Division of the National Psychological Association (NPA) entitled "Psychoanalysis Revised by War. Ethics, clinics, and Personal Experience" (October 2022), the joint conference of the European Association of Psychotherapists and the Ukrainian Union of Psychotherapists "Ethical Challenges for Psychotherapists in Our Changing World" (February 2023), the conference the Psychoanalytic Psychology and Psychotherapy Division of the NPA "Ethical Challenges in Psychoanalytic Practice in Wartime" (April 2023), and other events provided space for recognizing and addressing the gaps between the ethical codes and intrusive reality of war.

This chapter summarizes the ethical challenges that Ukrainian psychoanalytically oriented specialists discussed at the aforementioned events or in papers. It provides brief commentaries regarding the common ethical principles and specific ethics-related topics most affected by war.

Neutrality and Abstinence

Departures from non-interference and neutrality principles have become the most challenging and frequently discussed aspects of war adaptations among psychodynamic practitioners. First, as a psychoanalyst and an analysand found themselves in a joint catastrophic reality of war (Nalyvaiko, 2023a), it stressed the very possibility of being calm, accepting, neutral, and open to uncertainty for both of them (Romanov, 2023b; Velykodna, 2023a). With time, as Kokoilo mentioned, the war-related traumatic experiences of a psychoanalyst and an analysand were accumulated and often resulted in a situation where both of them met in the session being on edge (in Velykodna et al., 2023a). Many psychodynamic practitioners shared that they had doubts about whether to continue working, being overwhelmed with their psychic response to war (Romanov, 2023b; Velykodna, 2023b), and some of them decided to stop and refer their patients to colleagues (Lazos, 2023). How to continue working, knowing that you cannot be neutral and containing even if you wish to – that was the question.

Second, the invasion of Ukraine in 2022 was accompanied by new waves of Russian propaganda in which the war was both denied and glorified (Krishnarajan & Tolstrup, 2023; Romanov, 2023a; Zaleskyi, 2023). These extreme experiences (e.g., war exposure, intentional lies, and gaslighting) and reactions to them (such as fight, flight, or freeze responses) on the one hand, and frightening news about the success of the propaganda on the other hand (which managed to attract some of Ukraine's citizens to help Russian military with directing missile strikes and seizing some territories more quickly), required more than just recognition from analysts, but also unambiguous commenting and, often, open discussion of the patient's and analyst's actions and decisions for survival (Velykodna, 2023a). In these circumstances, those who attempted to look neutral and avoid discussing their attitude to war and its consequences by redirecting patients' inquiries into questions or interpretations were perceived as suspicious and dangerous as potential supporters of the war (Velykodna et al., 2023b).

Moreover, abstinence occurred to be something that threatened the analytic process and the therapeutic relationship not only imaginary but real. When, in the face of approaching war atrocities, the patient engages in self-soothing or self-blaming for wanting to escape instead of rescue, and the analyst remains abstinent, there is a risk that one from the analytic dyad would literally die. As Butenko-Hachkivska noted, psychoanalytic practitioners need to look for new ways of implementing ethics in wartime because the "ordinary ethics" with its primacy of respect for any decisions of the patient might pose a risk for psychoanalysis potentially serving the death drive in wartime (in Velykodna et al., 2023b). That is why Ukrainian psychoanalytic practitioners felt required to move away from the usual stance of abstinence, shifting more to crisis and supporting mode (Dorozhkin, 2023; Pustovoyt, 2023). It included various manifestations, for example, providing crisis interventions (Fedorets, 2023), sharing evacuation information and discussing evacuation plans, providing sessions free of charge (Nalyvaiko, 2023b; Rudenko, 2023; Velykodna, 2023a), reaching funds to provide patients with social and financial support (see Iryna Valiavko's presentation in Velykodna et al. (2023b), etc.

No less critical were rearrangements regarding the setting, considering the war and the imposition of martial law. The psychoanalysts were those responsible for discussing new rules for psychoanalytic sessions and payments in case of air raid alerts or other intrusions of war (e.g., during the months of regular blackouts due to missile strikes on the electrical grid, analysts and analysands often were unexpectedly unavailable for remote sessions). Such rearrangements included, for instance, suspending the sessions in case of air raid alerts when the analytic dyad met in person or when the alert was on the patient's or analyst's location only, without paying or with partial paying in this case. There were cases when, during their remote sessions, a patient did not inform the analyst about air raid sirens in their city because they wanted to continue the session. Suddenly, the analyst heard explosions from the patient's side through the zoom. These and other cases are moments when we believe the analyst is obliged not to show acceptance and tolerance of excessive risk and not to be abstinent or neutral. These are cases in which it is necessary to respond very clearly:

> I, too, value our sessions very much. I, too, look forward to meeting you and get disappointed when the meeting is canceled due to a missile attack. However, because these sessions are important to me, I insist that you take your security, and therefore, our sessions could continue even if some sessions are interrupted. But the sessions cannot continue if you die.

In sum, ethics, designed to create security, in warfare time requires the analyst to shift from neutrality to the declaration of an expressed ethical statement (including support or confrontation regarding what is good and what is bad in the topic offered by a patient when the patient showed their need in such recognition) while maintaining the analytic stance simultaneously (i.e., by refraining from unnecessary suggesting analyst's thoughts, beliefs, attitudes to the patient which was not a demand). This task was often perceived by Ukrainian analysts as an unresolved ethical dilemma (Nalyvaiko, 2023b). During peacetime, psychoanalysts usually have enough time to think about an intervention, consult with colleagues, and search the literature for clues. In times of war, analysts were often in a situation where they had to make a decision rapidly, which was often choosing among several bad options (Velykodna, 2023a). However, being an analyst also means being a human who upholds universal human values, sharing and support of which can be more important than any analytic identity in times of universal upheaval (Pustovoyt, 2023). In a war situation, the survival of two people and the survival of relationship between them were considered more important than adherence to the ideals of psychoanalytic practice.

Self-Disclosure

Independently of their psychoanalytic background, practicing approach, and attitudes to self-disclosure – whether it was previously seen as an obstacle for the transference development or a legal instrument of supporting the therapeutic alliance – the war forced Ukrainian psychoanalysts to face the impossibility of being not self-disclosed (Lagutin, 2023; Nalyvaiko, 2023a). First, patients witnessed – live or through the media – what was happening in the city and country where the analyst was located. Similarly, when the analyst fled the permanent location because of war, but the work continued remotely, this change in the analyst's life also became obvious to the patient (Velykodna, 2023a). As meeting with analysands at the analyst's home is not common in Ukraine (using offices in psychological centers or psychoanalytic institutions is more widespread), sometimes, patients began to ask in which district of the city the psychoanalyst lived to limit their fear about his or her life, i.e., not to be unnecessarily frightened when the news spoke of explosions in other districts of the city. Of course, at other times, such apprehensions might be interpreted in terms of the patient's phantasies regarding the analyst's death, but in a situation of being overwhelmed by the topic of death, not providing such information was felt as a mockery of the patient who was trying to ever so slightly improve their mental condition. Therefore, analysts were more open to direct answers to such direct questions, as well as to asking similar questions, clarifying what the analysand does during an air raid alert, etc.

Second, as aforementioned, patients sought certainty regarding the analysts' attitude to war. They searched for this information on social media or asked directly during sessions and in correspondence (Velykodna et al., 2023b). If the therapist responded in a non-disclosing manner, trying to maintain their pre-war psychoanalytic stance, it provoked anxiety and was perceived as a threat and as unsafe, which often led to interruptions (Dorozhkin, 2023). However, there is also another danger of this situation – when a patient knows (rather than fantasizes) about the psychoanalyst's attitude toward the war or his or her personal involvement in it, and this attitude does not coincide with the patient's own; the risk of interrupting therapy in this case also increases significantly (Lagutin, 2023). When the analytic dyad survived, a psychoanalyst's attempts to avoid self-disclosure by rejecting their own experiences within the session and interpreting the patient's feelings formally from an ordinary analytic stance looked like indifference to the patient while acknowledging the existence of similar experiences was more appropriate to the patient's need to be accepted and understood (Lagutin, 2023).

In general, the therapists' voluntary or involuntary self-disclosure inevitably influenced the content of the sessions and the transference development, to a certain extent making it possible to express various emotions toward the figures of the Big Others (disappointment, resentment, anger, pride, suspicion) and to accept the therapist's castration (i.e., non-omnipotence) and, through it, their own castration as well (Dorozhkin, 2023).

Non-Exploiting of Transference

As the previous parts of this paper reveal, there were many situations in which psychoanalysts were required to exploit the patient's transference. For instance, when the patient was stuck in a regression (relevant to the phase of psychoanalysis but irrelevant to the demands of escaping war) and the transference created a false impression that the psychoanalyst's omnipotent love to the patient is stronger than a real-life threat (i.e., nothing should be done, you are saved because you are connected with this exclusively good object), we believe it was crucial for the analysts to leverage this transference to let the patient survive, for example, by fleeing the territory about to be occupied by Russian troops.

At the same time, as Turbina (in Velykodna et al., 2023b) warns, psychoanalysts should be sensitive to their ability to refrain from using their transferential power and attacking the patients' way of experiencing the war. Referring to the factors that challenge the subjectivity in wartime (the destructive nature of war, the intense large group dynamics, and ubiquitous ideological propaganda), described by E. Levinas (1961), she indicated that in these circumstances, it is often difficult for analysts to distinguish between real and historical truth of analysands. The reason is that they, like their analysands, are themselves captured by the abovementioned factors. Thus, some psychoanalysts appeared to be tempted to promote what they consider a real truth for the analysands instead of exploring the patient's thinking and perceiving when there was no necessity to do so for survival. As a means of preserving their own subjectivity and their ability to listen analytically to the analysand by allowing them to reveal their own subjective truth, Turbina suggests that analysts seek a stance described in her metaphor of the "keeper of the keys in the temple." Within this stance, a psychoanalyst should only open the door to the "temple of psychoanalysis" and assist the analysand in encountering their own inner meaning, which is the goal of psychoanalysis.

Being especially aware of the importance of non-exploiting transference was also associated with the observed inversion of the therapeutic relationships perceived by patients: seeing their therapist in a vulnerable position, the analysands offered various kinds of assistance (including sending money and housing), becoming the "adult" in the therapeutic couple and turning the therapist into an object of care (Dorozhkin, 2023). As Dorozhkin (2023) noticed, these offers, though developed with a good purpose of preserving the invested object and the analytic dyad, often masked disappointment and grief because of the loss of the parenting object in their transference.

Confidentiality

In wartime, confidentiality was violated in several ways. First, as Saliy remarkably described (in Velykodna et al., 2023b), our patients tried to come to their remote sessions from any available places where often it was simply impossible to have privacy: bomb shelters, staircases in building entrances, train stations, bathrooms, because they had no other options. On the one hand, this expressed a great deal of trust in the analyst and an investment in therapeutic relationships and psychoanalysis, as well as their need for support. However, on the other hand, psychoanalysts have had to accept the risk of breaching confidentiality, for which we normally bear full responsibility. We have dealt with this issue like doctors assessing which would do more harm: to intervene or not to intervene in these circumstances. And leaving patients alone by declining to provide sessions because the changed reality of the patient's life did not fit the standard setting was considered more potentially harmful than risks related to confidentiality.

However, other breaches of confidentiality took less of the patient's benefit into account. For example, some psychologists, including psychodynamic specialists, reported cases (e.g., disguised or composite ones) in social media or to representatives of the media or authorities to illustrate the terrible crimes committed by Russian troops (Velykodna et al., 2023b). These reports were justified by the purpose that the world should know about the terrible crimes of Russia and also by the fact that the patient did not mind sharing the case. For some time, all those who openly spoke the truth about something were perceived as brave heroes and fighters for the truth. Nevertheless, the story, which did not become a complaint to the police and was not proven, is legally just gossip. At the same time, societally, it caused panic and horror in the population, as some people experienced the news of the reported cases as secondary trauma. It was felt that trust in psychotherapists as they tell the whole country about their patients has been undermined. The ethics committees of the associations began to process collective complaints from other psychologists about such cases.

Among the most vulnerable groups who suffered because of violations of confidentiality were children. As Zaleska reported (in Velykodna et al., 2023b), cases of child therapy, illustrated by their photos, drawings, and other materials, were especially wanted among journalists and funds who sponsored Ukrainian NGOs to provide therapy for free. Journalists were interested in telling painful stories to a national and an international audience to testify to the brutal consequences of the Russian invasion and show the resilience of Ukrainians and the courage of therapists in working with these issues. Foundations and non-governmental organizations needed stories and photos as evidence of their essential work, including to collect new donations and provide even more assistance to Ukrainians. In fact, children and their parents had to pay for this therapy by allowing the violation of the confidentiality of their participation in the project. Many therapists lost their previous patients because of the war, which means they lost their jobs. Therefore, working for an NGO, they found themselves in a vulnerable, dependent position and often could not resist the demand of the organizers to provide photos or drawings of the children they treated. To resolve this issue, Zaleska proposed asking children to use their drawings or texts, discussing the purpose of it, and making photos from the child's back to conceal the face and, thus, to avoid breaching confidentiality (in Velykodna et al., 2023b).

Professional Competence

Professional competence is the basic requirement for conducting psychoanalytic practice. In Ukraine, various national societies affiliated with distinguished international associations for psychoanalysis and psychotherapy provide full psychoanalytic training and continuous education (Nalyvaiko, 2023c; Romanov, 2024; Velykodna, 2025). However, faced with the need for psychological assistance within the population from the very first days of the 2022 Russian invasion, Ukrainian psychoanalysts often had no time to consider whether they were educated or experienced enough to provide crisis-related care, having on their backs only a basic psychoanalytic training. Although many psychodynamic specialists have been involved in crisis interventions since the 2014 Russian invasion of Ukraine (Fedorets, 2023; Pustovoyt, 2023), these experiences were rarely integrated into training programs. Some therapists attended short courses from Ukrainian and foreign experts in crisis interventions and actual trauma care and then went straight to work. Moreover, many psychoanalytic training programs were paused due to the war, but candidates often had to start their practice to address the war-related issues that became prevalent in the society (Velykodna, 2023b). Only later, as Arshevska-Guérin described (in Velykodna et al., 2023b), there appeared opportunities to discuss the observed effectiveness of psychoanalytically-informed crisis work in purposely developed new supervision groups and conferences, and Ukrainian psychoanalytic specialists began to summarize their experiences, make recommendations and focus on questions that have not yet been answered.

As Saliy (in Velykodna et al., 2023b) highlighted, during the war, the psychoanalysts should refrain from trying to work in the classical psychoanalytic manner using either silence or interpretation, which they have learned. Instead, Saliy suggests that we adapt psychoanalytic work to the needs that arise in crisis, using the concepts and techniques of holding (Winnicott, 1960), containment (Bion, 1963), and emotional reflection (Kohut, 2009). These concepts provide a working framework that helps to reduce tension and build greater trust between analyst and analysand, which is particularly necessary in a time of war. Using post-Lacanian ideas, Khrystenko (2024) recommends that psychoanalysts use therapeutic mediation through art in their practice. Therapeutic art ateliers can help revive psychic activity, overcome inhibitions, reform symptoms, and sometimes even strive for "synthome" in Lacan's terms (Lacan, 1976). These are only several topics that could enhance psychoanalytic education programs.

Working in wartime also showed some "blind spots" and disadvantages of ordinary psychoanalytic training. First, psychoanalytic practitioners often had insufficient knowledge of the evidence base of their approach, including the effectiveness and efficacy of working with crisis, actual trauma, and its consequences (Velykodna, 2025). It also resulted in that governmental and non-governmental mental health support services did not have data on the effectiveness of this approach and did not include it in their programs.

Only in December 2023, the situation significantly changed due to several publications regarding psychoanalysis as an evidence-based practice in the *Ukrainian Psychoanalytic Journal* and negotiations with Ukraine's Ministry of Health Care, which finally included the section of psychodynamic psychotherapies into a list of methods with proven efficacy.

Second, most psychoanalytic specialists were more proficient in the ethical norms established for the psychoanalytic method to maintain an asymmetry of therapeutic relationships and the analytic stance, in contrast to the general ethical requirements for mental health professionals and Ukrainian laws relevant to working with people. For instance, many psychodynamic professionals were unaware of the limits of confidentiality set by law, not by the method (Velykodna, 2023b). Similarly, certified specialists often had no idea how their practice should be legally formalized or what contracts for working with individual patients or with NGOs looked like. We believe these are essential questions that should be covered in the curriculum of basic psychoanalytic training.

Self-Care

The incredible tension experienced by psychoanalytic specialists in the described conditions of life and work emphasized the particular role of self-care as a means of maintaining a therapist's mental health and practice, including for vicarious trauma prevention (Velykodna, 2023b). Self-care became the subject of analysis and discussion, especially regarding the ethics of work during the war. As Medynska noticed, in wartime, psychoanalytic therapists should consider the specific exhaustion of their ability to mentalize, contain, and bear the intensive phenomena of the sessions, which she termed "material fatigue" similar to the process described in physics (in Velykodna et al., 2023b).

Fortunately, most Ukrainian psychoanalysts demonstrated developed safe-care skills, which allowed them to seek help and additional education, take care of themselves, and refrain from risky behavior (Velykodna, 2023b). A good knowledge of their unconscious helped specialists not to fall into the trap of inner processes that are dangerous during war. For example, those who usually live on credit funds began to show greater frugality. Those who liked to drink stopped or significantly reduced their alcohol consumption. Those who tended to rely on untrustworthy others took more responsibility for themselves. These are just some of our observations.

Many Ukraine-based and international professional societies offered Ukrainian psychodynamic specialists support groups, therapy, and supervision projects. Professional societies focused on crisis and trauma mitigation provided Ukrainian psychologists with various training, including developing self-care skills. These activities not only supported psychoanalytic thinking but contributed to a life drive and were perceived as therapists' self-care activities (Yevlanova, 2023). This international support allowed Ukrainian specialists to help others (i.e., patients, colleagues, and loved ones) while taking care of the analysts themselves.

Relationships with Russian Colleagues and Patients

To date of the full-scale Russian invasion in 2022, many Ukrainian psychodynamic practitioners had patients, analysts, and supervisors located in Russia and were involved in various joint activities with them, such as advanced training. The issue of maintaining or suspending professional relationships with them as Russian residents arose from several perspectives. First, from the very beginning of the invasion, many Russians, including psychoanalytic specialists, appeared to be either open war supporters or those who denied the existence of the invasion (Benvenuto, 2022; Romanov, 2023a; Yakushko, 2023; Yevlanova, 2023). This circumstance significantly changed the shade of cooperation with them as it is difficult to support the link with the other without the feeling of the *shared reality* in which red is red, war is war, and the victim is the victim.

What could usually be described in terms of an encounter with the tolerable otherness of other people has turned into facing an enemy that represents a threat to one's life. This raised the question of the extent to which psychoanalysts can tolerate and bear otherness in this situation. For instance, when the Russian patient says to the analyst, "I support the fact that my country seeks to seize more territories, including yours," of course, we should remember the individual psyche and the transference. Hence, we could elaborate our hypotheses about the desire to capture the analyst and even about a positive dynamic where the patient, perhaps for the first time, appropriates their aggression and greed in this identification with the country. However, in the context of the real war, it was difficult for Ukrainian psychoanalysts to bear the feelings caused by war, both in life and in practice, even when it was conducted with people who had also suffered from war or were against this invasion (Kechur & Haber, 2023; Romanov, 2023b; Velykodna, 2023a). The tension that arose in analytical and professional relations grew excessively, and the risk of acting out and enactment increased (Lagutin, 2023). Therefore, the question arose whether it is ethical for Ukrainian practitioners affected by war to pretend that they are ready to contain this otherness in relation to the sides of war conflict considering the risk of abusing the Russian patient, trainee, or supervisee (who does not necessarily but could take up arms and literally become an enemy) for their origins, political preferences and propaganda influence as well as for their unconscious dynamics manifested through war topics.

In contrast, some Ukrainian psychodynamic practitioners received valuable support from friends, patients, and colleagues from Russia and wanted to maintain these connections but feared condemnation for doing so. Members of the ethics committee and the head of the Psychoanalytic Psychology and Psychotherapy Division received a range of questions regarding whether Ukrainian specialists have the right to personal and professional contact with Russians in these conditions. Soon after these issues appeared, the government of Ukraine officially prohibited all kinds of economic, educational, and public relations with the residents of Russia as potentially dangerous collaborations. This decision additionally forced psychoanalytic practitioners to suspend their treatments and other activities with Russians, which was not always easy (see the brief report on such suspension authored by Yulia Melashchuk in Velykodna et al., 2023b); however, questions regarding personal or non-monetary collaborations still required the answers.

In response to this inquiry, an all-Ukrainian working group was organized with the representatives of most psychological societies led by the International Addiction Psychotherapy Association aimed to prepare a resolution regarding relations with Russian psychologists and psychotherapists in wartime (Velykodna et al., 2023a). Following this resolution, Ukrainian professional societies suspended any forms of cooperation with Russian psychologists and psychotherapists and their associations, regardless of their civic position and political beliefs, until the end of the war and appealed to their members with a request to refrain from professional contacts with Russian psychologists and psychotherapists, while personal contacts were distinguished as not covered by this document. Last but not least, the ethics of public discussion of political leaders (in particular, Vladimir Putin) by psychoanalytic specialists was elaborated with an emphasis on the need for such publications but with a warning about the limitations of their conclusions (Kechur, 2024; Lupis, 2024).

Conclusion

Overall, the ethics of psychoanalytic work during the war was transformed by special attention to the threat of the destruction of connections (intrapsychic and interpersonal) in order to support the life drive and invest in the trust and dignity of the patient. The dehumanization that characterizes military invasions permeates many areas of life and relationships. Preservation and creation of psychoanalytic relationships and attempts to resolve the ethical dilemmas which occurred supported counteraction to dehumanization and restoration of humanity.

Finally, it is worth mentioning Winnicott's (2021) idea of a "good enough mother" who never knows what her child needs exactly but tries to understand and sometimes succeeds in it. Similarly, Ukrainian psychoanalytic professionals faced various ethical questions to which they did not know the answers. However, we assume that the fact that they tried to find the appropriate answers, including by discussing them with colleagues and dealing with patients ethically enough in this impossible time, contributed to the fact that psychoanalytic work succeeded in continuing in many cases.

References

Benvenuto, S. (2018). *What are perversions?: Sexuality, ethics, psychoanalysis*. Routledge.

Benvenuto, S. (2022). Psychoanalysis in the war. A debate with Russian colleagues. *European Journal of Psychoanalysis*. Issue 'Lights Ablaze from Ukraine and Russia'. https://www.journal-psychoanalysis.eu/articles/psychoanalysis-in-the-war-a-debate-with-russian-colleagues/

Bion, W. R. (1963). *Elements of psycho-analysis*. Heinemann.

Burka, J., Sowa, A., Baer, B. A., Brandes, C. E., Gallup, J., Karp-Lewis, S., … & Rosbrow, P. (2019). From the talking cure to a disease of silence: Effects of ethical violations in a psychoanalytic institute. *The International Journal of Psychoanalysis*, 100(2), 247–271. https://doi.org/10.1080/00207578.2019.1570218

Butsykin, Y. (2023). Translating psychoanalytic texts into Ukrainian: Discoveries and further steps. *Psychoanalytic Psychology*, 40(4), 261–265. https://doi.org/10.1037/pap0000483

Crastnopol, M. (2021). Doing what's right: The ethical dimension of psychoanalytic work during a pandemic. *Psychoanalytic Perspectives*, 18(3), 362–373.

Dorozhkin, V. (2023). Current war and its impact on the therapeutic relationship. *Ukrainian Psychoanalytic Journal*, 1(1), 32–35. https://doi.org/10.32782/upj/2023-1-6

Fedorets, O. (2023). Counseling on the front line: Insights from a Ukrainian doctor. *Psychoanalysis, Self and Context*, 18(3), 345–351. https://doi.org/10.1080/24720038.2023.2209129

Filts, O. (2023). Evolution of psychotherapists' ethics before the war and during the war. Presentation at the conference *"Ethical Challenges for Psychotherapists in Our Changing World"*. https://youtu.be/7LhGCvFIyzw?si=vM4XS_eo6ef62ykO

Goodman, D. M., & Severson, E. R. (Eds.). (2016). *The ethical turn: Otherness and subjectivity in contemporary psychoanalysis*. Routledge.

Harcourt, E. (2015). The place of psychoanalysis in the history of ethics. *Journal of Moral Philosophy*, 12(5), 598–618.

Kechur, R. (2023). Ethics of freedom and ethics of totalitarianism. *Presentation at the conference "Ethical Challenges for Psychotherapists in Our Changing World"*. https://youtu.be/mZf0QOAuKnE?si=o9CbbfX7gQOSonVi

Kechur, R. (2024). War. Individual or collective madness? A commentary on the "Leadership analysis in international affairs: A psychodynamic perspective" by A. Lupis. *Ukrainian Psychoanalytic Journal*, 2(1), 118–121. https://doi.org/10.32782/upj/2024-1-13

Kechur, R., & Haber, D. (2023). An exchange with Roman Kechur: Preserving thinking during wartime. *Psychoanalysis, Self and Context*, 18(3), 364–378. https://doi.org/10.1080/24720038.2023.2203028

Khrystenko, O. (2024). Graphic interpretation as an instrument of therapeutic mediation of subjective time ordering. In the example of a clinical case with a psychotic patient. *Ukrainian Psychoanalytic Journal*, 2(1), 67–76. https://doi.org/10.32782/upj/2024-1-8

Kohut, H. (2009). *The analysis of the self: A systematic approach to the psychoanalytic treatment of narcissistic personality disorders*. University of Chicago Press.

Krishnarajan, S. & Tolstrup, J. (2023). Pre-war experimental evidence that Putin's propaganda elicited strong support for military invasion among Russians. *Science Advances*, 9, eadg1199. https://doi.org/10.1126/sciadv.adg1199

Lacan, J. (1976). *Le Séminaire, livre XXIII* (1975–1976). AFI.

Lagutin, V. (2023). Psychoanalysis "traumatized" by war. Four clinical illustrations of the vulnerability of the setting. *Ukrainian Psychoanalytic Journal*, 1(3), 18–23. https://doi.org/10.32782/upj/2023-3-3

Lazos, G. (2023). Transformation of psychotherapeutic relationships during the war. *Psychoanalysis, Self and Context*, 18(3), 382–387. https://doi.org/10.1080/24720038.2023.2203158

Levinas, E. (1961). Totalité et infini (Vol. 19652). The Hague: Nijhoff.

Lupis, A. A. (2024). Leadership analysis in international affairs: A psychodynamic perspective. *Ukrainian Psychoanalytic Journal*, 2(1), 108–117. https://doi.org/10.32782/upj/2024-1-12

McWilliams, N. (2020). The future of psychoanalysis: Preserving Jeremy Safran's integrative vision. *Psychoanalytic Psychology*, 37(2), 98–107. https://doi.org/10.1037/pap0000275

Merlino, J. P. (2006). Psychoanalysis and ethics—Relevant then, essential now. *Journal of the American Academy of Psychoanalysis and Dynamic Psychiatry*, 34(2), 231–247. https://doi.org/10.1521/jaap.2006.34.2.231

Nalyvaiko, N. (2023a). Borders and psychoanalysis in a time of war. *Psychoanalytic Psychology*, 40(4). http://doi.org/10.1037/pap0000485

Nalyvaiko, N. (2023b). Ethical transgressions in psychoanalytic practice during the ongoing war. *Ukrainian Psychoanalytic Journal*, 1(2), 19–23. https://doi.org/10.32782/upj/2023-2-2

Nalyvaiko, N. (2023c). *Psychoanalysis in Ukraine. History. Present. Future.* Akademia.

Palii, V. (2023). Ethical aspects of psychological work in Ukraine: Past, present, and future. *Ethics and Behavior*, 33(3), 220–230. https://doi.org/10.1080/10508422.2022.2152030

Pustovoyt, M. (2023). Interpreting crisis while in crisis (reflections on psychoanalytic work in hybrid warfare). *Ukrainian Psychoanalytic Journal*, 1(1), 21–26. https://doi.org/10.32782/upj/2023-1-4

Rajchman, J. (2013). *Truth and eros: Foucault, Lacan and the question of ethics*. Routledge.

Romanov, I. (2023a). Contemporary propaganda and propagandistic states of mind. *Ukrainian Psychoanalytic Journal*, 1(3), 24–29. https://doi.org/10.32782/upj/2023-3-4

Romanov, I. (2023b). The war inside: Unconscious experience of war in a patient and an analyst. *KnotGarden*, 2, 67–85.

Romanov, I. (2024). Geschichte eines ukrainischen Psychoanalytikers. Mein und unser gemeinsamer Weg. *Psyche*, 78(6), 508–534.

Rudenko, R (2023). Traveling through the worlds: New challenges in therapy with children, adolescents and their families during the war. *Psychoanalytic Psychology*, 40(4). http://doi.org/10.1037/pap0000481

Velykodna, M. (2023a). A psychoanalyst's experience of working in wartime: On choosing between bad options. *Psychoanalytic Psychology*, 40(4). http://doi.org/10.1037/pap0000480

Velykodna, M. (2023b). Russia's war against Ukraine and some issues of psychoanalytic training. *Ukrainian Psychoanalytic Journal*, 1(1), 47–53. https://doi.org/10.32782/upj/2023-1-8

Velykodna, M. (2025). War and attacks on thinking: Reflections on the Psychoanalysts' responses to the 2022 Russian invasion of Ukraine. *Psychoanalytic Inquiry*, 45(4). https://doi.org/10.1080/07351690.2024.2355172

Velykodna, M., Arshevska-Guérin, O., Davoian, Y., Dorozhkin, V., Manzar, V., Monakhova, N., & Khrystenko, O. (2023a). Resolution on regulating relations with Russian psychologists and psychotherapists during Russia's war against

Ukraine. *Ukrainian Psychoanalytic Journal*, 1(1), 66–68. https://doi.org/10.32782/upj/2023-1-11

Velykodna, M., Nalyvaiko, N., Pavlovska, O., Arshevska-Guérin, O., & Butsykin, Y. (2023b). Ethical challenges in psychoanalytic practice in wartime: Conference report, Kyiv, Ukraine, 2023. *Psychodynamic Practice*. https://doi.org/10.1080/14753634.2023.2258036

Winnicott, D. W. (1960). The theory of the parent-infant relationship. D. Winnicott, (1965). *The maturational processes and the facilitating environment* (pp. 37–55). International Universities Press.

Winnicott, D. W. (2021). *The child, the family, and the outside world*. Penguin UK.

Yakushko, O. (2023). Psychoanalysis and war: Histories of resistance and support for war violence. *Ukrainian Psychoanalytic Journal*, 1(1), 14–20. https://doi.org/10.32782/upj/2023-1-3

Yevlanova, E. (2023). Professional supervision as therapists' self-care during wartime. *Psychoanalytic Psychology*, 30(4). http://doi.org/10.1037/pap0000486

Zaleskyi, D. (2023). The war of symbols. Symbolization and identity in the context of Russia's war against Ukraine: Analytical view. *Ukrainian Psychoanalytic Journal*, 1(3), 30–34. https://doi.org/10.32782/upj/2023-3-5

Chapter 7

Effects and Affects of War in Psychoanalytic Practice

Oleh Khrystenko

Ethics and Metapsychology of Working with Affects in Times of War

War is the ethical opposite of psychoanalysis. The war forces human beings to move toward death while fighting for their lives within the deathly war. Human beings cannot avoid the deformation of the symbolic order that protects from the invasion of the real or from everything that cannot be symbolized. In the formulation of a Ukrainian psychoanalyst Velykodna and colleagues (Velykodna et al., 2023),

> It can be said that psychoanalysts have a reputation as advocates of aggression no less than advocates of sexuality. However, the symbolic realization of aggression means that the subject refrains from real action, deed, an act in a state of affect, which satisfies the aggressive urge, replacing them with words and fantasy, purposefulness, and legal competition. In the context of the life of civilization, there are three fundamental rejections related to aggression, which mark the transition from animal to human: rejection of murder, incest, and cannibalism.
>
> (p. 66)

War brands the analytical process as fragile, but the analytical process is also perceived as a cure for war, directed in the opposite direction of war—toward life. As I formulated earlier (Khrystenko, 2021),

> Psychoanalysis is directed towards life regardless of the paradigm. The Lacanian maxim "do not give up your desire" is interpreted by me above all as faithfulness to lack, which lies at the heart of desire, and from there, faithfulness to the movement of life. There is another aspect of faithfulness to desire. Let us recall Antigone. Antigone died, but she was

DOI: 10.4324/9781032660257-8

> on the side of Life because she preserved human dignity, refusing the whim of the tyrant; she preserved her inclusion in the symbolic order. The ethics of other psychoanalytic paradigms are also linked to being on the side of Life. Freudian loosening of demands, Id and the Superego, which is a culture of the death drive — is a stance in support of Life. In the verdant Green of psychoanalysis, binding of drives, objectalization, and subjectalization — isn't it a movement towards the triumph of life? Integration of the personality, as an ethical position of the Kleinian psychoanalyst — doesn't it lead to the victory of life over destruction? The ethics of psychoanalysts — to be on the side of Life. In the flourishing realm of Green's psychoanalysis, binding of drives, objectalization, and subjectalization – is it not a movement towards the triumph of life? Integration of the personality, as an ethical position of the Kleinian psychoanalysis, does it not lead to the victory of life over destruction?
>
> (p. 113)

The ethics of psychoanalysts is intended to be on the side of Life.

The war has become a catalyst for a more active transformation of psychoanalysis-oriented practices. Ukrainian psychoanalytic psychotherapist Valeriy Dorozhkin (2023), analyzing the trends of war, concludes that the transformation of psychoanalysis amidst war is, in fact, accomplices a more humane and open approach. In my practice, I have found this transformation in numerous ways, but especially in an emphasis on working with my patients' affective states.

Certainly, before the war, affective states were always centrally present in my practice. Although I might not have followed the so-termed classic psychoanalytic formulations, I paid attention to representations of the affect in the unconscious and suggestions by André Green (Green & Weller, 2012). In my opinion, Green's theorizing about affectivity and emotions in human experience is an important contribution to psychoanalytic clinical practice.

On the other hand, formulations of what constitutes affect are also common in psychoanalysis. Lacanian psychoanalyst Colette Soler (2012) suggested:

> The term "affect" — in German, Affect with a "k" — was popularized in psychoanalysis by Freud, who took it from an earlier German philosophical tradition, where this word denoted a pleasant or pathological state along the lines of satisfaction and dissatisfaction… The ambiguity

> of the term is interesting in that it was applied both to the body and to the subject.
>
> (p. 6)

Affect, therefore, is viewed as the companion of drive, human desire, and human needs.

The affects are directional. Specifically, the following considerations of its presence in human functioning were suggested initially by Freud (1915): (1) displacement or regression toward a psychosomatic phenomenon; (2) the suppression, restraining affect; (3) the transformation of affect into anxiety, when non-utilized libidinal energy transforms into fear.

From this theorizing, psychoanalytic clinicians can view the task of an analytically oriented clinical work as accompanying the patient in the interaction with affective states. In psychoanalysis, the affect by its nature, like the drive, is situated between the human soma and the psyche. The affective states must also arise from excitement, for which the Other serves an originating function. Thus, one of the goals of psycho-practice is to accompany the subject in transforming undifferentiated excitement into affects. Another aspect of psychoanalytic work is found in the integration of various ways of negated affect back into conscious states. The return of true representation of affect, the liberation from suppression, and so on are also key parts of the practice.

In psychoanalytic-oriented practice, it is important to bring back the affect to where it belongs—from the unconscious to the conscious—in order to prevent the impact of trauma from forming isolated fractured affective states that are likely to re-emerge in the form of suffering and symptoms. This work must be perceptive and sensitive because it is important not to overload the patient with what cannot be borne, preventing mental disorganization.

The painstaking return of affect is ethically defensible because it serves Life—the force that integrates negated, displaced, and suppressed affects. Through such efforts, the analyst might prevent pathological repetition, which can occur when the psyche is incapable of integration.

The Effects of War

In my view, the central effect of war is the distortion of the symbolic order via the intrusion of the real, that which cannot be inscribed into the symbolic and imaginary registers. This real cannot be shielded by the usual screens. This real is experienced as excessive excitement that cannot be represented. In Nalyvaiko's (2023) summary, "Trauma is something that, by definition, is not represented. Therefore, the analyst's task at this stage is to help the analysand to construct a verbal, through a signifier, defense against the intolerable Real" (p. 29). In war, we surmise, human beings experience a reduction of drives and affects into excitement. When drives cannot manifest themselves in objects, they turn into painful dissatisfactions. There is a tragic unraveling of the drives of life and death. Through the search for signifiers in war, human beings unravel the veil of the imaginary and symbolic, protecting themselves as subjects from the intrusion of the real. Theoretically, it is difficult to neglect the imaginary register or its reintegration; this process becomes technically appropriate in times of war.

The second effect of war is found in a torrent of losses. The stability is lost. The predictability is lost. When close relatives and acquaintances die from war violence, human beings face losses in their worst forms. However, witnessing the deaths and losses of others is also traumatic. Social connections are disrupted as people move within the country or emigrate abroad. A Ukrainian psychoanalyst Natalia Nalyvaiko (Nalyvaiko, 2023) noted in her published diary:

> The first month of the war was a month of total losses: material and immaterial—homes, jobs, all our past identities. Our belief in fundamental human kindness was undermined, our sense of security in this world was destroyed, and trust was betrayed.
>
> (p. 27)

Analytic relationships were often impossible to maintain, and the analytic process was not always physically possible. For some of us, it became psychologically impossible to withstand the deluge of traumatic affect, especially when repetition, compulsion, and significant transference emerged in unprecedented ways. For other people, the analysis psychologically saved them.

The third effect of war is found in the emergence of narcissistic trauma. We often witness the ruins of normal neurotic narcissism, which, for most people, serves as the preserver of life. Normal narcissism is found in harmony between libidinal investment in oneself and in the external world. It helps enrich the self through intersubjective connections that leave a mark on the intrasubjective and help maintain personal uniqueness. This normative narcissism is the guarantee of self-development and a sense of self-love as well as self-respect. During the war, the movement of libido between external objects and the Subject becomes distorted. Sometimes, I observe de-objectalization, when the external objects are no longer saturated with libido, leading to Subjects' boredom, ruptures in relationships with others, and neglect of the ordinary aspects of their life. In other cases, de-subjectalization occurs when subjectivity becomes disinvested of libido, sometimes manifesting as a silent decline in personality or in attempts to satisfy endless demands. This process often leads to hatred directed toward the world, which becomes the barrier to their Ideal-I. For many analysands, the fact that war has occurred in their own lives and in their country's life was a narcissistic injury because they thought such a thing could never happen to them. In other cases, their own Self is attacked blamed as the culprit for misfortunes and, leading to melancholic distress. In my practice, I worked with cases of analysands who were convinced that the outcome of the war depended personally on them: that if they could work persistently enough, they could ensure victory and peace. Certainly, his process turned into self-hatred because invariably, they realized their limitations in the face of current events.

The third path for many individuals seems to be found in the sublimation of suffering and its elevation toward greater goals, which often make life bearable for many analysands and gives meaning to their lives. In this case, it is important not to take away this development but also to return the persons toward themselves and their lives in order to establish a certain balance.

The fourth effect of war is inhibition. The most common complaint I hear in analysis during my work today is a decline in vigor. Most often, patients describe this as an inhibition that is associated with the work of grief. This grief often has a specific object of loss—a loved one killed in bombings or the death of a partner who served in the military. However, frequently, such an object has a diffused characteristic, and even the neurotic psyche finds it difficult to identify and articulate. Moreover, most people live within the condition of constant micro-traumas that cannot be processed in time, leading to increasing inhibition of the psyche. Occasionally, the psyche is inhibited by unconscious desires that conflict with a person's values, leading to aggression toward society or government or a desire to return to past lives at any cost. In the case of losses, an analytically oriented clinician seeks to articulate them and initiate grief work, while, in case of unwanted desires, to understand them.

The fifth effect of war is found in the transition from the level of desires to the level of needs. Although Lacan (2011) insisted that in psychoanalysis, we should work with desires instead of needs, it is often irrelevant in work during wartime. As Lacan demonstrated in his seminar *Desire and its Interpretation*, even the level of needs is coded into the realm of the human creation by the great Other, ensuring that needs become a component of a cultural order. During war times, however, human needs are impossible to ignore or avoid because they have universal human relevance. René Roussillon (2023) conceptualized further the needs of the Self, which are necessary for the Self to perform its work of integration, mentalization, objectalization, and subjectalization. Roussillon identified two main clusters of the needs of the Self: safety needs and transformation needs. Safety needs include predictability, the importance of sharing affects, and creating meaning (Roussillon, 2023). Psychoanalytically oriented work can partially meet these needs and compensate for their deficit in reality. War is the very definition of uncertainty and unpredictability, while the structured, organized setting and the availability of the clinician help patients compensate for the chaos of reality. Intrusion of what cannot be symbolized at a particular moment in a patient's life can gain symbols in analytical practice, achieved by transforming excitement into affects and words. The analysis becomes a space for meaning-making and the recognition that not everything can make sense without devaluing life.

By fulfilling the need for safety, the human psyche can move on to the need for transformation. These are the needs that facilitate the transformation of excitations into psychic representations and make life in the body and external reality sufficiently comfortable. Like the safety needs, these requirements are also heterogeneous. They are possible as a consequence in relation to an external object. Transformation needs depend on the object and its characteristics. For transformations to occur, the object must be psychologically available and susceptible to influence, be sensitive and capable of adapting to needs, not be destroyed by the influence of destructive forces, retain the memory of encounters with the subject, be consistent, and not be disorganized. These characteristics in an analytically oriented clinical work must occur within a therapy setting, which is vital during the turbulent times of war as prerequisites for symbolization.

The Affects of War

The primary affect people encounter during the war is anxiety. Anxieties exist on different levels. According to Bergeret (1974), three levels of anxiety within three structures of the psyche are recognized. In a neurotic structure, the castration anxieties are typical. For borderline states, separation anxieties are prevalent. For psychotic structures, the anxiety of disintegration prevails (Bergeret, 1974). As analysts we encounter these anxieties both in peacetime and during wartime practice. Remarkably, Freud's (2014) differentiation of anxieties became relevant to me in reading his work *Inhibitions, Symptoms, and Anxiety*.

The object of anxiety is either an excess of knowledge or found in its lack. When the war began, Ukrainians encountered a deficit of information. Many people, including myself and many of my patients from the Kyiv region, on the first day of the war found themselves in a situation of total uncertainty when it was unclear how to leave the city, whether it was possible to leave, whether Russian troops were already inside the city and whether it was safer to elsewhere versus hiding in the basements. On the first day of the full-scale invasion, I could not get to my office, but the internet still worked, so I switched my practice to a remote format. All of my analysands were scared, but fear elicited different reactions in everyone. The foremost difficulty, however, was the literal impossibility of planning either the next sessions or life itself. Safety needs were brutally violated. My decision was to preserve what was possible, which in our case was access to me and analytic treatment. Thus, from that day on, I offered everyone to work online as much as possible and under as safe conditions as we could create. The economic uncertainty arose, so with some patients, new prices were set while others continued to attend at the old rates but in the form of credit. For some patients, it was important to maintain the prior session fees despite any changes in their lives, so we chose payment in hryvnias (Ukrainian currency) but in an amount equivalent to the euro exchange rate at the time of the invasion. Thus, even payments for each session provided the insurance of certain safety. Safety became the condition for reducing anxiety. The main focus of the sessions at that time was on symbolizing anxiety. Typically, we talked about day-to-day experiences, but sometimes we linked them to transference or the past, but the latter were exceptions to the rule.

In the following days, I lost my internet connection, and I could not leave my home because it was near the front lines. The only thing I could accomplish, albeit with difficulty because of unstable cellular connections, was to send text messages stating that I had to cancel sessions indefinitely. I assured my patients that I would inform them of when I could resume our work and that they were welcome to seek alternative psychological assistance during this time. Thus, I attempted to convey that despite my current unavailability, I would resume work when it was possible and that I desired to continue the analysis as well as to be the same person they approached for analysis originally. However, if a patient's condition was particularly complex, I stressed and ensured that they sought help from other clinicians.

The most challenging aspect of working during wartime, eloquently described by Ukrainian psychoanalyst Volodymyr Lagutin (2023), is "the loss of the ideal asymmetrical situation for the analytic process, where the patient is inside the trauma while the analyst is outside. In this case, both are engaged in the common experience" (p. 19). The safety needs of both parties in the analytic process are destroyed. While in peacetime, the analyst can consistently provide a safe space through the facilitation of a setting, in wartime, analysts find themselves amidst unpredictable events and often experience effects and affects that are similar to those of their patients.

It is important to return to considering the variety of anxiety conditions that I worked with during wartime. Freud (2014) distinguished three main groups of anxieties. The first one is related to the fear of losing parental love, the second is—the fear of punishment, and the third is connected to the fear of being rejected by society. The fear of losing parental love was not frequently activated by the war in my practice, although this anxiety itself is common in my analysands. However, at times, this anxiety was activated among some patients. For example, one analysand found it extremely challenging to talk to her mother on the phone because her mother moved from Ukraine to Russia ten years prior and held relatively pro-Russian sentiments. In our work, other memories of their parental relation were stimulated when her mother's object merged with the image of the attacking "Mother Russia," including the fear of experiencing aggression, including my aggression, toward her mother.

The fear of being excluded from society, which is one of Freud's initially noted anxieties, was also present in this analysand, and was discovered through her dream. In one of our sessions, she recalled a dream about her colleague "Lesya," who became insane and attacked their acquaintance, whose surname was that of a well-known Russian writer from Kyiv. Free associations led her to conclude that "Lesya" represented Ukraine because, above all, for the analysand, "Lesya" was the famous Ukrainian poet Lesya Ukrainka (2014), whose work focused on the liberation of Ukraine from Russian oppression at the turn of the 20th century. In her association, the analysand herself was her colleague because she was of Russian descent, like the writer whose surname she dreamt. Moreover, in everyday life, the analysand communicated in the Russian language (i.e., many Ukrainians were Russified, reflecting centuries of Russian imperial practices). As it turned out, her associations led her to recognize that she was afraid of being excluded from Ukrainian society and that she feared it would attack her for being "different." She also felt guilty because of her identification with Russians, which she feared made her complicit in attacks on Ukraine, so therefore she projected aggression into Ukraine's response. This fear of punishment manifested in her life in later sessions. This analysand was forced to flee to Western Europe, where she initially found relief from her anxiety. However, after a month, she began experiencing problems that could be traced to her own defenses. For example, she procrastinated in processing her refugee documents, complicating her life while also constantly discussing irrational fears about other's responses to her. Gradually, we began to work through these fears and anxieties caused by her feelings of guilt because she felt relatively content in W. Europe while Ukraine was burning under Russian attacks. She again feared punishment for this happiness, and she brought punishment upon herself.

Among forced Ukrainian migrants, both within the country and abroad, nostalgia is widespread. Nostalgia is one of the consequences of a disrupted need for safety, specifically the need for stability. In this situation, it acts as an analgesic, helping people to escape from painful reality into a world of fantasy about recognizable stability, where a person feels safe and protected from failures in their actual lives. Moderate nostalgia also connects the past with present reality, providing a continuity of life experience. Nostalgia is a manifestation of necessary investment in objects of loss, which is essential for beginning the work of mourning. However, prolonged nostalgia can indicate an inability to grieve because those and that which is lost can destructively overshadow the present. Thus, nostalgia can have both vital and mortal manifestations. When it aids in mourning work or contributes to a sense of life's continuity, it aligns with Eros. However, when it competes with reality when it is a manifestation of de-objectalization, it aligns with the death drive. In the former case, we simply accompany our analysands, while in the latter case, we either intensify the work of mourning or work with analysands as we do with melancholic patients.

Often, alongside mourning work comes boredom. There is everyday boredom when people find themselves at a crossroads in their object relations. However, there is also pervasive boredom, which is a manifestation of melancholy. This pathological boredom is the result of deep disappointment, when unconsciously people expected something delightful, via unprecedented pleasures or paradisiacal delights yet these objects do not exist. The longing is experienced in the form of uncontaminated pressure toward nowhere, and thus, the longing cannot find satisfaction. In Lacanian theorizing, this is "jouissance," which Juan-David Nasio (1998) described as the pressure that arises in the erogenous zone of the body, which seeks to reach a certain goal, which encounters obstacles on its way, which seeks an outlet and then accumulates. The jouissance is tension without satisfaction (Nasio, 1998). Jouissance can manifested via various accompanying affects, such as boredom. Boredom connected to jouissance is overcome by accepting limitations. For example, one analysand felt dreadful boredom after she focused on victories of the Ukrainian army as the primary object of her satisfaction. However, when the frontline areas of Ukrainian defense were slowed, she felt pervasive boredom and irritation. In overcoming this boredom, the analysand had to acknowledge that there is no ideal object that can always provide satisfaction, that satisfaction itself is always limited, and that the idea of endless pleasure is only an impossible illusion. This path of mourning encompassed both her current situation and events of the past, as well as her infantile fantasy of unlimited parental satisfaction.

Often in our work we encounter hatred, usually directed toward perceived offenders. However, hatred can also be the result of envy. One of my analysands takes pride in her husband's volunteer military service, although she noticed that she could not communicate with her best friend. She had several dreams about herself in the role of an aggressor, harming her best friend. Notably, her unconscious hatred was born out of envy because her friend's husband did not join the military and was safe and seemingly enjoying normal civilian life with her friend. This recognition sparked a desire to destroy her friend's pleasure, but her love for her friend did not permit her to acknowledge this feeling. Thus, as a compromise, she simply could not continue her relationship with her friend, although this friend appeared in her dreams.

Most of the affects of war are experienced as profoundly unpleasant. Space for other affective states also must be found amidst the war. People experience joy when they discover that their friends were unharmed despite the drone hitting their house. There is space for love directed at loved ones as well as for your city, for your Motherland, and for the best of humanity. Most importantly, there is the possibility for hope, which is also nurtured in psychoanalytic spaces because this hope is not built on the negation of reality but hope that is rooted in the essence of human existence. This hope is the basis for survival in difficult times and the aid we need to endure suffering. The foundation of such hope is found in the ability to be creative. It is found in overcoming emptiness and futility, which is connected to perceptions of the world as rigid or unchangeable. Hope is located in the belief in change, in the belief that pleasure is possible, even if these cannot be present now. Hope is the ability to rely on self internally. It is the belief that the world is potentially good and that it is merciful. This belief is based on the deepest strata of the human psyche, which is often related to primary caregivers, who often came back to us in time and transformed the pain of separation so it could be endured. If this experience is connected to the foundational aspects of psychic function, then a person indeed can have hope. At times, this hope saves us during chaotic events that otherwise could only evoke despair. If the positive experience is not rooted in the psyche, then the world is doomed to turn into hell. Such encounters can then be based on love, solidarity, religion, art, and (notably) in psychoanalytic practices.

References

Bergeret, J. (1974). *La personnalité normale et pathologique* (Vol. 2). Dunod.

Dorozhkin, V. (2023). Current war and its impact on the therapeutic relationship. *Ukrainian Psychoanalytic Journal*, 1(1), 32–35. https://doi.org/10.32782/upj/2023-1-6

Freud, S. (1915). Instincts and their vicissitudes. *Standard Edition*, Vol. 14, 109–140.

Freud, S. (2014). *Inhibitions, symptoms and anxiety*. Read Books Ltd.

Green, A., & Weller, A. (2012). *Key ideas for a contemporary psychoanalysis: Misrecognition and recognition of the unconscious*. Routledge.

Khrystenko, O. (2021). Psychoanalysis in person and online: Ethics, discourse, frame. *Psychoanalysis and the virtual: Ethics, metapsychology and clinical experience of the remote practice: Conference proceedings*, June, 12–13.

Lacan, J. (2011). *The seminar of Jacques Lacan: Book VI: Desire and its interpretation: 1958–1959*. AFI.

Lagutin, V. (2023). Psychoanalysis "traumatized" by war. Four clinical illustrations of the vulnerability of the setting. *Ukrainian Psychoanalytic Journal*, 1(3), 18–23. https://doi.org/10.32782/upj/2023-3-3

Nalyvaiko, N. (2023). Language metamorphoses as representations of subjectivity. Ukraine. Dairy of war. *Ukrainian Psychoanalytic Journal*, 1(1), 27–31. https://doi.org/10.32782/upj/2023-1-5

Nasio, J. D. (1998). *Five lessons on the psychoanalytic theory of Jacques Lacan.* SUNY Press.

Roussillon, R. (2023). *Manuel de la pratique clinique en psychologie et psychopathologie.* Elsevier Health Sciences.

Soler, C. (2012). *Les affects lacaniens.* Essaim.

Ukrainka, L. (2014). *The Babylonian captivity.* (Trans. S. Newborn). Mudborn Press.

Velykodna, M., Arshevska-Guérin, O., Davoian, Y., Dorozhkin, V., Manzar, V., Monakhova, N., & Khrystenko, O. (2023). Resolution on regulating relations with Russian psychologists and psychotherapists during Russia's war against Ukraine. *Ukrainian Psychoanalytic Journal,* 1(1), 66–68. https://doi.org/10.32782/upj/2023-1-11

Chapter 8

War-Forced Terminations of Psychoanalysis

Cases from Ukraine

Mariana Velykodna

The new Russian invasion of Ukraine in 2022 encountered psychoanalysts with various expected and unexpected difficulties (Romanov, 2023; Velykodna, 2023). In addition to the obvious issues of defense and survival, psychoanalysts and their patients had to deal with both the threat of forced interruption of their work and the risk of disruption of previously planned terminations of psychoanalysis. Talking about interruptions, I do not mean solely that sessions could not continue (Nalyvaiko, 2023). Of course, in wartime, many analytic dyads were separated, including by death or forcible displacement. Numerous analyses were stopped or paused without the possibility of even saying goodbye. Dozens of specialists suspended their practice in response to war (Lazos, 2023). However, many analyses succeeded to continue, even in circumstances close to impossible (Lagutin, 2023).

In this chapter, I focus on cases when war forced or highly impacted the termination of psychoanalysis. However, in my view, it still could be seen as a termination, not an abrupt withdrawal or rupture. In part, the presented cases show that war itself can set a particular transference line where the analyst is seen as victimized, vulnerable, betraying, or even a destroyed object with whom it becomes impossible to grow up. My observations taught me that in such situations terminating may be the right decision if it symbolizes an active refusal of this dynamic and supports the life drive. Another line in presented cases maintains the role of meaningful decisions to oppose the power of meaningless events in external reality. Along this line, termination could be seen as a support for subjectivity instead of obedience to fate. Overall, the proposed cases may illustrate the margin between traumatic loss set by war (as abrupt disappearances, disruptions, and abandonments) and ordinary loss (which can be accepted, processed, and mourned)

DOI: 10.4324/9781032660257-9

required for terminations of psychoanalysis. They highlight the extreme difficulty to provide the patients with appropriate termination in wartime.

The Pre-War Setting of My Psychoanalytic Work

Before the 2022 Russian invasion of Ukraine, I worked partly in person at my office in Kyiv and partly online with Ukrainians and people from other countries of the former Soviet bloc (e.g., Belarus, Estonia, Latvia, Lithuania, Russia), including migrants from these lands all over the world. My practice encompassed psychoanalytic work with neurotic and non-neurotic (in Andre Green's terms; Green, 2018) patients in various (intensive and non-intensive) settings. One can notice in the described cases that some of them are more likely to be called therapy or even psychoanalytically informed interventions, while others are closer to ordinary psychoanalysis. This well reflects my practice in general, which is evidence-informed and responsive to a patient's specifications and life setting. Regarding termination, in all cases, we had an initial agreement not to make abrupt withdrawals but to discuss the termination process and the desire/need to leave.

Terminations in Wartime: Clinical Illustrations

The proposed cases were chosen as illustrations of three different aspects of war's impact on the terminations of psychoanalysis that I have faced with my patients since the 2022 Russian invasion of Ukraine. I am grateful to all the presented patients for their consent to be published in this book and for their feedback on my drafts about them.

I also wish to let the reader know that in all these cases in 2022, I had limited time and capacity to think and choose the best available option (as I have already described in Velykodna, 2023), and my supervisors were not available during that period. Therefore, the cases reflect the decisions and offers that I could make rapidly in the described conditions to support the logic of termination instead of an abrupt and traumatic loss.

Case 1

The first case concerns a young woman located in a Muslim country who was studying psychology and was inspired by lectures on psychoanalysis, which led her to seek analysis. I will call her Maria. Maria's childhood was spent in one of the countries of the former Soviet bloc. Her parents, like other people at that time, had difficulties with housing and first lived with Maria's mother's parents. Maria remembers this time fondly, which seems to have been largely supported by her grandmother but gave the impression of a very close and loving family overall. Around the age of 3–4, she and her parents moved to a new house in a different city. During that time, the family lived separately, the parents' relationship deteriorated rapidly, although Maria did not notice it then. At age 6, her mother suddenly packed up and secretly moved away to another man's house together with Maria. For some time, she was asked to lie to her father over the phone and say that they were visiting her grandmother and would return soon. She felt like a betrayer of her father and was very sympathetic to him.

About six months later, the secret was revealed, and Maria wanted to spend all her free time with her father, not her mother and stepfather. She came to her father after school and on weekends. Gradually, she had to recognize that her father was an alcoholic and did not take care of the household at all. Later, it turned out that this was the case from the very beginning and was the reason for her parents' divorce, but Maria was not told about this for a long time and did not understand it. Instead, she thought for a long time that her father was just sad because they had left him. She tried to do her best around his house and hid the alcohol. Every day, her father came home drunk, and she had to take care of him and put him to bed. Sometimes his condition was so bad that she was afraid he would die. It was only in her late teens when her father started a new relationship, which again failed because he had an alcohol assumption, that Maria realized that her father was using her or other women as housewives and lifeguards, not really wanting to change himself.

When Maria entered college, she felt that she wanted to start a good family with a man who did not drink alcohol. She took this issue very seriously. When she learned that men of the Muslim faith are not allowed to drink, she decided that she would convert to Islam to find a mate. Soon enough, Maria met a Muslim man whom she chose with her mind rather than her heart. She liked him for his serious willingness to create a family and to work hard, although, at that time, he was quite poor and worked as a part-time taxi driver. She supported him in every way possible and helped him to eventually develop a successful business.

When we met, Maria was the mother of four children and she was drowning in housework. Despite the fact that her husband had a good business and Maria helped him with it, the family lived very frugally. Her husband was reluctant to spend money on the family, and Maria herself could not insist on her needs. Maria took on a part-time job as a counselor to pay her bills. She felt unnecessary and unappreciated in her marriage. She was also worried that her husband might take a second wife. Her usual way of building relationships since childhood, through serving others, caring for them, and supporting the household, had come to a standstill. She also discovered that her children were taking on their father's pattern of abusing Maria's care. The consequence of this long history was the development of a specific sacrificial thinking, in which there was no place for the recognition of her own attitudes, thoughts, and desires. Her studies in psychology and lectures on psychoanalysis made her question why she had chosen this man and this relationship, this religion, and the denial of her own needs in favor of the needs of others.

We worked online twice a week using a couch for over two years. It was an interesting and productive work on reconstructing Maria's family history, including various difficult events and processes, her present life, and her sexuality. During these two years, Maria was able to work through her deep guilt over her father's fantasized betrayal, which she has been atoning for all her life, as well as the painful triumph of being his only love when the mother left him. During the therapy, Maria began to live a more active social life, changed the family's financial and household arrangements, started a new education, and began to express herself more as a full partner in her husband's business.

Whereas before, in a situation of frustration, her thinking seemed to be inhibited, and she experienced frightening bodily experiences and fantasies, now Maria used her thinking freely and creatively. She was also able to make decisions and act on them. Most notably, when others acted in an infantile and irresponsible manner, Maria could now confront them instead of rushing to cater to them. As a therapist, I was happy with this dynamic and proud of her general success. Once, we discussed with her that the initial request for therapy had been met, but she shared that her professional identity required the continuation of psychoanalysis in order to have a place to talk and think about herself.

The outbreak of the war in Ukraine significantly interfered with the described dynamics. Maria was terrified and wept all the time, thinking about me. Her daily routine and plans were suddenly interrupted. Although I left Kyiv on the first day of the invasion and lived in the west of the country for about a week, in a safe place, and then went to Poland,[1] Maria was inconsolable. She felt incredibly sorry for my war exposure and forced displacement and felt that she both wanted to and could not help me. She shared fantasies about Marie Bonaparte, who gave all her money to save Sigmund Freud during WWII. And she reproached herself for not being able to make such a great gesture for me. At our sessions, she shared that she could not talk about herself because I was in such a terrible situation. She also noticed with pain that she wants to continue analysis, although she hardly tolerates the sessions now.

I felt that we were at the heart of a process where a father (me in transference) is in a severe condition because of alcohol (because of mother's and daughter's betrayal—as Maria thought), possibly dying, and his little daughter is trying to do something out of an agony of guilt and powerlessness. This is a girl who could not live the life of a child because neither her mother nor her stepfather nor her father himself intervened to tell her: "It's not your responsibility, and it's not your fault. You don't have to deal with it. This is for adults to figure out." Neither of these adults forbade the girl to spend so much time with her alcoholic father, with whom she had no care and was at much risk as if she were completely alone. It seemed that this heavy dynamic was destroying everything we had been building for two years. In the transference, I became a figure of her care, as Dorozhkin (2023) described it. But I would add that it was a figure of impossible care because she could not objectively help me but was unable to mentally accept this impossibility as well.

After several attempts to interpret this process, which were unsuccessful in comforting her affects, I felt that in order to preserve the gains that psychoanalysis had already made for Maria, an appropriate adult finally had to appear in the process. My impression was that it was not solely a word but a psychoanalytic act that was needed to stop this "jouissance" in Lacan's (in Braunstein, 2020) terms. Referring to the line of transference and her father's history, I told her that I had known for a long time that there would be war here, but I chose to continue living in Ukraine. And now, it is my own decision to leave the war zone for the time needed. Yes, these are difficult events for anyone, but I can handle them; I am not destroyed, and I am going to keep protecting my life. So, I said, I am grateful to Maria for her compassion, but there is no need and no obligation for her to deal with this tragedy that has befallen my country. There are other adults here who are handling the situation.

I also added that these devastating events in Ukraine, similar to other tragedies, should not destroy *everything* around. We had a fruitful work for more than two years, many good things were discovered or created within this process. And if the war and having an analyst affected by war threatens the whole analytic progress and everything good Maria obtained in it, we should stop here to preserve what was achieved. It was the first time Maria stopped weeping and her steady breathing resumed with every word I said. I felt that this was a good moment to also remind her that her father must have said something similar: "No, this shouldn't destroy you. This is something that happened only between me and your mother. And it is my decision to deal with it *like that.*" Maria replied after some pause that she had a strange, very distinct feeling as if I had said something very right, which she experienced in her body as calm and correct, although she had never allowed herself to think about termination before.

We had two more final sessions, during which Maria was already in a calm state, in which great gratitude, as well as regret and sadness, were expressed in turn. She discussed how much had happened in the analysis already, and we both recognized that we had not expected to stop now, but we should. She reminded me of the most valuable changes and achievements she associated with this therapy. And we ended by feeling that it was a forced but correct decision to terminate psychoanalysis in order to *preserve* the psychoanalytic work that had already taken place.

Case 2

My second case was conducted in person in Kyiv. With Natalia, an intelligent and talented woman of about 40, we worked in a classic format of three sessions per week using a couch for five years. In Natalia's initial address, many topics were about the pain of abruptly leaving relationships. It seemed that she had not yet grieved the divorce from her ex-husband, which happened almost a decade ago, but was experiencing the pain of new breaks: with men, friends, therapists, and other missed opportunities.

Natalia's childhood memories were almost devoid of pleasant things. One of the earliest refers to the second year of life when she was taken from her father's arms because she was admitted to a children's hospital for a week. At that time, in the Soviet Union, parents were prohibited from being together with their children in a children's inpatient hospital. Since then, she has been stuttering for a long time but has never been to a speech therapist.

Regret settled in her parents' home very early on. It is not known for certain what was the root cause of regret. However, Natalia remembers that it was the feeling that the relationship between her mother and father had been in the process of being destroyed, though no one talked about it directly.

When the girl was 6 years old, her very handsome and successful father once took her to work with him, where his female colleague hinted to Natalia that they would soon live together. This woman was indeed her father's lover and became his wife many years later when Natalia became an adult. This event in her childhood also added to the feeling that something was slowly collapsing and that it was impossible to overcome. One remains to live in impossible mourning for an event that has not yet happened. At the age of 13, Natalia first heard from her mother that her father was asking for a divorce. Since this topic had been kept quiet for years, the girl responded very vividly that it would be great if her parents could finally get a divorce. However, she received a slap on the wrist from her mother. Her parents waited to divorce until Natalia grew up, although her father had a parallel relationship with another woman all his life and later married her. All of this created an impression of the unloving mother (which was, to some extent, transferred to women in general) and of the over-valued father and men in general.

In adulthood, when Natalia faced something that made her dissatisfied or disappointed in relationships, she often was as if paralyzed by these dynamics and waited for the collapse instead of taking action, such as seeking constructive solutions through conversation or conflict as well as deciding to separate by herself. The collapse was always near. And then, in the aftermath, she could long for this relationship as an idealized good one. And all the parts that were not remembered as good were explained with pain as Natalia's fault. During the years of psychoanalysis, Natalia often worried that I would leave her. At first, these were fears expressed indirectly. For example, she might think that my belly looked like a pregnancy. Or she had a fantasy that my husband might accidentally meet and flirt with her (like her father, who flirted with many women in front of her eyes). Sometimes she made it clear that the analysis did not give her anything: I was still perceived as smart and successful, but she was not. And these thoughts were connected to the painful idea that I would abandon her (as I hypothesized—because of her wish to identify with me and her fear that it would seem too competitive and unbearably aggressive for me).

At some point, it became clear that all of Natalia's object aggression (ranging from envy and a desire to incorporate and be identified with—to dissatisfaction with being mistreated) was turning into masochistic suffering and an attempt to prolong a bad relationship to preserve the object at least a little good. For this task, she alternately unconsciously identified with her mother and the lover of her father, both of whom were attached to him. However, both these identifications seemed unhappy. This pattern also posed a real danger to her health, as it was used even in her relationships with doctors. If a doctor failed to help, Natalia could not simply go to another doctor. Instead, she would continue treatment that didn't work, then quit, but keep going to the same doctor until they said they couldn't help.

In our work, we have largely analyzed these patterns and Natalia's fantasies about phallic others (men or married women) and the "defects" that lead to abandonment by these others. Within these fantasies, for a long time, there was no equal pairing, no ending that was not abandonment. When I first asked Natalia how she envisioned the termination of the analysis (around the beginning of the third year of therapy), she was afraid of this question and, as she later admitted, began to prepare for a collapse—that I would soon leave her. Her experience of the early trauma of being left in the hospital and the emotional atmosphere in her family were constantly reproduced in her adult life, including in psychoanalysis. Gradually, through the analysis of her history, current events, and the enactments in the analysis, we were able to disclose these fantasies and see the high price Natalia pays for maintaining these images. It was important to restore her right to want what others have, to identify with them, and to change objects and desires. It was also important to allow herself to identify with the one who was leaving, abandoning, and competing. In this process, she realized that she wanted to abandon her career and become a photographer, like a classmate she met by chance.

By the end of 2021, we had spoken a lot about what good endings to relationships between people can look like. This topic gradually touched upon psychoanalysis. At the time, she felt stuck in the sense that it was a valuable experience, but the thought of its ending was stealing the joy of each session. So I suggested that we try to discuss and clearly plan the termination of psychoanalysis as something that would happen at a mutually agreed time that would take into account her needs and give her enough time to process. After some thought, she said she liked the idea of ending in nine months, in the summer of 2022. We also discussed what she wanted to say or do during that time and agreed with this date.

The Russian invasion in February 2022 challenged these plans. Each person in Ukraine faced their own mental response to this event, often reactivating previous traumatic experiences. In Natalia's case, it was about triggering feelings of helplessness, abandonment (as many of her friends and I had fled the city), and disorientation. Her work as a photographer stopped, and Natalia had to live on her savings, which would not have been enough for psychoanalysis sessions. The first thing I did was to offer her to continue our sessions online as agreed but without the usual payment. Instead, if she had time and resources, I suggested that she do some charitable help for others, which would be a symbolic payment for the sessions (as Francois Dolto (1985) suggested). She gratefully agreed. Our sessions at that time focused on containment of Natalia's feelings and discussing her hesitations about whether or not to leave the city and the country, whether or not to look for another job, and whether or not to ask others for help. She felt calmer when her friends from different cities in Ukraine and abroad invited her to their homes. She did not go to them in the end, but knowing that she was not left to fend for herself provided tremendous support. Later, she found a part-time job as a photojournalist with an NGO that helped war victims, which also allowed us to return to paid sessions.

By the end of spring 2022, we were able to speak again about our plans agreed upon before the war. Natalia emphasized that the war had taken away so much and deprived her of so much that it was very valuable to her that we had kept our sessions going. Equally valuable was the fact that we could not passively succumb to the dynamics imposed by the war but follow our plans regarding the termination. At that point, we could ensure that each of us was all right and that termination did not mean leaving each other in trouble. In the summer of 2022, on the previously scheduled day, having managed to discuss the feelings, thoughts, and phantasies that accompanied this process, including mutual gratitude for this experience, we ended our therapy.

Case 3

The third case concerns Olga, my female patient from Russia, with whom I worked online for more than six years before the invasion. Olga had a significant experience of early trauma and abandonment, her first horrible memory dating to the age of three: her alcoholic father leaves her alone in a dark house to go to his friends until her mother comes home late at night. Other memories about Olga's childhood were about her mother, who, in my view, had an undiagnosed severe mental disorder that manifested itself in denial of reality and unlimited harming her daughters "for a good cause" (once Olga allowed me to listen to the recorded speech of her mother which provided confirmation of my hypothesis). And there often was no *third* to play the role of the father as someone who would limit the mother's abuse. The kind grandmother who visited and read her books and talked with her much during several months at the age of two was the only exception.

Despite her difficult childhood, which included her parents' quarrels, divorce, and, eventually, the death of her father, Olga managed to obtain a good education and develop many talents, especially in writing. She was married at a young age and had two children, but was disappointed in her husband and divorced him. When we met, she was an impressive mother of teenagers, divorced for the second time, and was seeking a new partner. However, she felt almost unable to cope with the challenges of life. She was plagued by procrastination and fears at work, despair in motherhood, disbelief in the possibility of change, and all attempts to establish stable relationships after the second divorce. In adulthood, Olga also experienced betrayal and persecution by significant others—lovers, colleagues, and acquaintances—which significantly undermined her trust in the world and in herself. For instance, humiliating bullying at work forced her to leave the good position she deserved. At some point, her recent and early painful experiences reached a state of acute trauma and dissociation, including panic attacks, which prompted Olga to seek psychotherapy.

Seeing me was her fifth attempt to start therapy after several that were interrupted for various reasons, mostly because the therapists abandoned her openly or latently (e.g., by abruptly doubling the price). Although Olga had previously tried to visit these therapists in person or online via video calls, at the time of her reaching me, she could not bear any meetings, being seen, described herself as feeling unnatural during meetings, and not able to express her feelings. So, she initially insisted that our sessions should be conducted in writing.

Since my psychoanalytic training was heavily influenced by Prof. Horst Kaehele, who always valued trusting patients and their symptoms and offering help that they can bear, I trusted Olga that we should start working online by correspondence, and from time to time, I mentioned that it would be good to try video sessions one day. This correspondence used a specific website for psychological assistance, where the patient and therapist or counselor had a confidential page for exchanging messages, similar to a forum. Having specific days and times for our written sessions, we worked this way for more than two years until our relationship became reliable enough for Olga to try video sessions. We quickly discovered that Olga's fears were justified—she felt extremely uncomfortable at video meetings, and many of her feelings and thoughts could not be caught and expressed during the session. To cope with this, we alternated between video and written sessions for another six months and, after this period, shifted to primarily video format of the sessions.

At the same time, the text of the writing sessions was stored, and Olga could return to these texts as a kind of transitional object (Winnicott, 2018) between sessions (which, as we both hypothesized, referred to her grandmother, who spent with her some time at the age of two). Sometimes, this object was comforting; sometimes, it was confusing. Sometimes, it was important to re-read something recent, sometimes something a year old, and sometimes the entire text of the therapy from the very beginning. Although some of my supervisors said that I was allowing something strange to unfold, it seemed important to me to analyze the meaning of these actions and relationships together with Olga but not to interrupt them or impose prohibitions on them. Besides, I saw many external indications that our therapy was helping Olga: she was engaged in an active job search and dating was directed at successfully finding a suitable partner.

Due to Olga's extensive traumatic experience, this therapy was not easy for either of us. She was very sensitive to the experience of abandonment, which was also reflected in our work. For a long time, she remembered with pain the few sessions I canceled. And no amount of apologies or explanations eased this pain. In addition, the experience of living with her mother, who constantly and deliberately distorted information, often brought new waves of distrust to our relationship, which she could generally trust. At the same time, it was obvious that Olga was making incredible efforts (mental, emotional, and financial) to keep this therapy going and to make it useful for her. She tried to explain to me in great detail what was happening to her and, if something had been acted out between us, how exactly I was involved in it. Sometimes her pain in contact with me was so strong that she asked for more written sessions instead of meeting on Zoom. In addition to protecting me from direct reproach by shifting her pain and anger into text, the transition to a written format allowed her to record our conversations, i.e., to collect evidence of what I had said or asked and to check if she understood and remembered me properly. In part, this protected Olga from a situation where I could deny something that happened during the video session as her mother often did. However, this storage of talks also assisted her in preserving a good experience. As I hypothesized, she used this text both as a good maternal object and as a fair father, *the third*, which exists in objective reality independently from our influence.

I sought a way to support her in this vulnerability, understanding that interpreting and analyzing her psychic experiences that unfold in a real therapeutic relationship and in transference, as well as just recognizing and containing them, is not enough. Once, during a video session, Olga tried to explain to me that I had said something unpleasant during our previous session, but I did not remember the episode well. She said reproachfully, "We should record you." I replied that it was completely acceptable for me to have our meetings recorded so that she could watch them in the same way as written sessions. We agreed that the recordings would be stored on a virtual cloud, i.e., equally available for Olga and me. Thus, she would be able to use them when needed, similar to the stored text. Our agreement regarding the video recordings included that Olga would tell me when she watched them so we could explore her needs or wishes associated with this action. This turned out to be a good decision, which helped our work a lot, both in terms of trust (by investing in a "fair father") and in developing a good object for incorporation, which is no longer just a text but a living person. In most cases, Olga needed to watch the recorded video when she had an unpleasant feeling after the session but could not identify exactly why it occurred. Watching the video allowed her to find that moment and watch it several times to explore her response and process her feelings, which she often could connect with her previous (including early) life experiences. Interestingly, after such a process that often included a kind of catharsis, Olga watched the whole video again, but she could then see it in a new way, and I was perceived more positively.

We worked in this way quite productively for almost a year when Olga first started talking about the possibility of ending therapy. At that time, Olga was involved in a positive, new relationship, even living with this new partner. Her children had grown up and started to live independent lives. Olga found a new job and was more confident in dealing with conflicts and life's challenges. I agreed that we could move toward termination, and we made slow attempts to decrease sessions and take longer breaks. However, with each attempt, Olga found that after a few weeks without sessions, she felt abandoned by me, despite knowing that it was our mutual decision to terminate. In addition, something painful or inexplicable at times came up in her life at these moments, and she felt in need of therapy. I assured her that we would stop when she was ready, so we went back to the sessions.

At the beginning of 2022, this slow termination process had been going on for a year and a half. In January 2022, Olga shared that she felt anxious at work, where she was recently promoted and was adapting to her new position. In the same period, it was already clear to me that the Russian invasion was inevitable. And, given Olga's experience of abandonment,

I was worried that I shouldn't disappear from her suddenly. I imagined that when the war started, I could be injured or lose electricity or the internet and not be able to let her know what was happening to me. On the one hand, I saw that her general functioning was better, and she was probably not so vulnerable anymore. But on the other hand, I was afraid of re-traumatization in the form of abandoning her in the face of a big and incomprehensible event. This prompted me to talk to her about a possible war and to agree that if I disappeared suddenly, she should know that I was doing everything possible to save my life and that I would get in touch when I could. During that conversation, Olga felt disappointed. She did not believe that such a threat was real and perceived my words as intimidating. She recalled her painful experience when her mother threatened her with suicide. In addition, it seemed that I had offended her by having negative thoughts about the country in which she lived. It looked to her that I was the one who attacked first. We worked through this conflict over several sessions.

Within a week, Russian troops entered Ukraine. The very first day I left Kyiv, I wrote to all the patients with whom I had a session that day or the next day, that I was on my way to a safe place and would write when I could offer to meet. Olga was among them. In the following days, we exchanged messages about the news a few times, mostly to keep in touch. It took me approximately two weeks to flee and settle in Poland, after which we were able to meet for an online session. Until that moment, it had already become known that both the Ukrainian and Russian governments had banned economic relations between our countries. Bank transfers were blocked, and contacts with the "enemy side" were considered illegal. This was the moment when I was forced to actually abandon this therapy, Olga, and, in fact, to betray our agreement. I was genuinely worried about how Olga would handle this moment.

However, Olga observed in herself an unusual new reaction to the cancellation of sessions. For the first time, she did not perceive my disappearance as an abandonment. Instead, she felt that there was something big and strong—*the third* (the war, the law, or authorities as symbols of paternal function)—that was separating *us*. And this separation was not as painful as previous ones. Olga felt pity, compassion, sadness, and concern about whether I was okay but not the well-known unbearable pain she had been living with for years. In several further control sessions, we summarized our therapy as well as discussed and accepted this specific moment when termination as a bearable loss could finally occur in unexpected circumstances, where *the third* separates *the dyad*, and *no one is abandoned.* Within the next two years, I received several very warm and touching letters about Olga's current life and her gratitude for the therapy we had, with light sadness that sometimes she misses it.

Beyond the Cases of Termination

Although the described cases are far from ordinary terminations and were affected by forced conditions, I recall Gabbard's (2009) warning that it is important to do our best to provide patients with just "good enough termination," not an ideal one (Kantrowitz, 2014; Shane, 2009). In my current commentary, I want to outline the key points I have tried to follow or learned from in these and other cases that were forced to be ended in wartime. As it has been two years since Russia's full-scale invasion of Ukraine and the events described, I still find it difficult to think in a normal way, my commentary on the cases described may appear superficial. I hope readers will be able to appreciate the difficulty I faced in dealing with forced terminations due to war as well as the challenges in my attempts to describe them, living in Kyiv during the ongoing war.

Termination and Its Criteria

Under "normal" conditions, termination is seen as determined by the internal logic of the psychoanalytic process, the patient's psychic forces, and the development of the analytical relationship. Freud (1914) distinguished termination from ending by the patient's ability to perceive the gains of psychoanalysis as their own, which he associated with the development and resolution of transference and related phantasies about the analyst's exclusive ownership of making analytic conclusions. In 1937, he broadened the criteria for termination by including the ending of the patient's suffering from initial symptoms, anxieties, and inhibitions and the analyst's assessment of the risk of their repetition as not likely (Freud, 1959). For a long time, the idea of termination, which referred to Freud's vision of psychic conflict transformation, remained prevalent (Brenner, 1976).

Later, termination tasks shifted their focus to the issues of analytic relationships, including attachment development, internalization and identification, acceptance of loss, and mourning (Orgel, 2000). The number of transference cycles during the analytic process was reconsidered as unconscious testing and efforts to develop and internalize analytic trust (Ellman, 1997). Using this lens, psychoanalysis was no longer of necessity defined as completed (Bonovitz, 2007). For instance, Shane (2009) believes that psychoanalysis should not terminate *everything* in analytic relationships as it may be potentially continued in the future:

> It [psychoanalysis] entails an important relationship evolving over time between two people, two people committed to one another, and who doubtless may come to love one another in the course of their work together. This is a kind of love based in profound and mutual respect, concern, and caring for the other's well being.
>
> (p. 168)

After such pleasant and valuable relationships have been developed, the patient needs enough time to obtain the capacity to think about termination (Holmes, 2011). This capacity is often associated with working through and mourning previous losses (Orgel, 2000). Another line in understanding good enough terminations considers the patient's learning from analysis. The best moment for termination could take place after a patient has already learned what it means to be both in an active process of analyzing and its metabolization between sessions, including vacations and other pauses (Schlesinger, 2013). In this case, the patient would value the discoveries of further self-analysis, even if the termination was processed in a form far from optimal (Zimmer, 2021). In sum, however, as Bergmann (1997) noted, psychoanalysts are rather guessing than knowing, which is the optimal moment for termination.

Termination Process

Knafo (2018) argues that termination need not be considered a distinct phase of the psychoanalytic process since we are dealing with loss throughout our lives and throughout our treatments. Some patients benefit from a long and defined termination period, while other do not; the second group feels more comfortable with spontaneously discovering the fact that their initial request for psychoanalysis was already addressed, at which time they feel they can stop coming (Shane, 2009). In contrast to the evaluation-focused criterion model of the termination period, attention to the patient's dreams, stories, and analytic dyad development, allows making terminations meaningful therapeutic acts (Grenell, 2002). I found it helpful to consider the following ideas formulated by Pediconi (2019), who also emphasized that termination is not mandatory associated with healing or being fully analyzed:

> ...termination rarely corresponds to a good outcome for a given experience, especially if the experience was complicated or distressing. But termination can be a good outcome when it *introduces a solution with satisfaction*. It remains a bad outcome when it involves a *suspension with pain or anguish*.
>
> (p. 35)

In my practice, I used to be guided by trusting my patients about their readiness or lack of readiness to terminate the analysis or take a break. But equally, I trusted my observations and conclusions when it seemed that the time for termination was not yet right for that patient. In such cases, I tried to explore and interpret the unfolding processes, but I always assured the patient that I would agree to a break if the patient needed one. My experience has shown that most patients who leave for a break come back. It often takes place after exploring their Oedipal dynamics and receiving the Oedipal promise—as a manifestation of their need in some *latent period*. Similarly, patients who have been working through childhood separation difficulties may want to take a pause to manifest and appropriate their separation freedom and then return no less freely, making sure that the relationship with the analyst is intact. In case of termination, I also trust the dynamics that unfold as quick and short or long and slow, which we can observe and discuss, being responsive to the phenomena of the very termination.

However, it would be naive to believe that one can offer terminations which would not be painful, as it always confronts the analytic dyad with loss. Even after the terminations that were perceived as good enough, 3/4 of the surveyed analytic candidates experienced mourning lasting from 6 months to a year, which was more difficult among those who had earlier traumatic losses in their history (Craige, 2002).

Termination in Wartime

In wartime, terminations, as well as continuations of psychoanalysis, are even more challenging. These tasks, often not easy in ordinary work, seem impossible or inappropriate amidst the war. Thus, as many analytic dyads faced the intrusion of war, we sought the minimal requirements to provide the analysands with a "good enough termination" in such circumstances. Here are some notes summing up my experience of termination in wartime.

Termination as Not the Only Option

Most importantly, I tried to continue therapy whenever possible. It often meant modifying the goals and the technique as well as changing the setting and format (e.g., Case 2). When war prioritizes excessive destruction, rupture, and death, I believe it is extremely important to resist this on all possible levels, including by maintaining connections and creating or protecting good things from destruction—i.e., supporting the life drive. And it significantly differs from conducting therapy in times of peace, when the reasons of forced termination are to be accepted, worked through, and mourned instead of resisting and seeking ways to hack them (Power, 2015). In my wartime practice, the main goal was to preserve psychic investments in good objects by surviving relationships invested in prior to the war. However, it was important to be aware of for whom I wanted to maintain this relationship: for my own sake or whether the analysand indeed needed it also (Skolnick, 2011). It also included a question of whether I am a good object for someone to invest in, as I am under fire or in the process of taking refuge. As my practice has shown (e.g., Case 1), sometimes the goal of supporting the life drive requires refraining from continuing psychoanalysis in such circumstances. Overall, the very ability to decide whether or not to end a treatment, instead of succumbing to the inevitable fate of war, is in itself a contribution to maintaining a sense of agency and subjectivity.

Inventing an Individual Transference-Related Termination Style

Unlike "ordinary terminations," when we expect transference to be resolved or comforted, in wartime, psychic functioning often reactivates previous conflicts, traumas, and issues regarding the relationships, even if they seemed to be resolved before. And it relates not only to war-exposed patients but also to those who became local or remote witnesses of war that affected a psychoanalyst. Therefore, observing the acute reactions of the patient to war, I tried to keep in mind the unfolding line of transference, as well as the key problematic points in the patient's history that could potentially be re-enacted. I tried to do so to base my hypotheses and decisions considering the previously gathered and currently perceived information. Generally, these were attempts to follow what Salberg (2014) described as seeking a good enough ending for each unique case. In Case 1, there was a risk for us to establish relationships similar to those that the patient had with her alcoholic father in her childhood and adolescence, which threatened the possibility for her to use her newly developed patterns in her own life. In Case 2, it was crucial to maintain work resisting the abrupt interruption of psychoanalysis while supporting the previously developed subjective decision on its planned termination simultaneously—as relevant to the core unconscious dynamics of this patient, who had been abandoned and suffered because of that. The third case also had a history of early abandonment and unclear communication with primary objects. Considering this background and our relationship encouraged me to talk with this patient clearly about the impending and, later, ongoing war and demonstrate my attachment and willingness to continue being connected while accepting its impossibility.

Seeking Meaningful Words for Meaningless Events

In my hypotheses and decisions, I tried to take time (when possible) and discuss the topics and options to continue (and how) or to terminate with the analysands, listening to what they thought and felt about it. In the cases in which termination was the best option, my goal was to find an optimal place and time for a mutual ending (Ellman, 1997) and to make a painful event potentially positively transformative (Lussana, 2018). Even when I had one session or less at my disposal, I searched for words that would limit the analysands' suffering, support them, and offer a symbolic pillar that would give our separation at least a little meaning, like in the presented Case 1. Sometimes this meaning was simply a recognition of the prematurity of the termination and sharing mutual regrets about it. Sometimes, it was an attempt to invest in the future. For instance, with my patients located on the territories occupied by Russian troops (for whom it was insecure to call me by phone or write messages) to keep hope alive, I could say that I would think of them and one day, when the madness of war is over or earlier, I would be happy to hear from them again and sincerely wish it would happen as soon as possible. When termination was inevitable due to the patient's location in Russia or Belarus, and I assumed that a real attack from their country on me would be a reason for these patients to feel guilty for the previous unconscious aggression against me, I clearly and kindly stated that I knew these patients were not involved in the war and my situation. If I knew that the patients often tended to experience themselves as betraying others, I tried to formulate clearly that they could seek another therapist nearby (i.e., allowing them to choose someone else if needed without guilt).[2]

Generally, if termination of psychoanalysis is inevitably perceived as loss (Orgel, 2000), in wartime, we should struggle to make it an "ordinary" loss for our patients and us (i.e., preserving positive aspects of treatment and transference) instead of a traumatic one.

Conclusion

Overall, the presented cases illustrate my efforts to transform the intrusion of war in a therapeutic process, which was perceived as meaningless, into at least partly meaningful decisions. This approach generally characterizes my psychoanalytic practice in wartime. I believe that this chapter illustrates my attempt not only to conduct a post-termination analysis of these cases (Zimmer, 2021) and to find a container for the unresolved issues (Grossmark, 2020) but also to continue them as if these cases can now survive within this book and the readers' minds in addition to my thoughts and my heart.

Acknowledgments

First, I would like to acknowledge my mentor at the Society for Psychoanalysis and Psychoanalytic Psychology (Division 39, American Psychological Association), Dr. Jane Hassinger, with whom we discussed the initial idea of this chapter through the cases presented during my Scholarship in 2023–2024. Second, I am grateful to Dr. Danielle Knafo, who provided valuable feedback to the final draft of this chapter and helped to improve it.

Notes

1 I am grateful to the people of Poland for the opportunity to receive temporary protection there. I stayed in Poland for six months and returned to Kyiv, Ukraine.

2 About a year later, I was happy to be acknowledged that most of my patients from abroad with whom we could not continue working for various reasons already found new therapists. It means for me that investment in good objects and processes survived.

References

Bergmann, M. S. (1997). Termination: The Achilles heel of psychoanalytic technique. *Psychoanalytic Psychology*, 14(2), 163–174. https://doi.org/10.1037/h0079713

Bonovitz, C. (2007). Termination never ends: The inevitable incompleteness of psychoanalysis. *Contemporary Psychoanalysis*, 43(2), 229–246. https://doi.org/10.1080/00107530.2007.10745906

Braunstein, N. A. (2020). *Jouissance: A lacanian concept*. SUNY Press.

Brenner, C. (1976). *Psychoanalytic technique and psychic conflict*. New York: International Universities Press.

Craige, H. (2002). Mourning analysis: The post-termination phase. *Journal of the American Psychoanalytic Association*, 50(2), 507–550. https://doi.org/10.1177/00030651020500021001

Dolto, F. (1985). Paiement symbolique. *Séminaire de psychanalyse d'enfants*, 2, 35–42.

Dorozhkin, V. (2023). Current war and its impact on the therapeutic relationship. *Ukrainian Psychoanalytic Journal*, 1(1), 32–35. https://doi.org/10.32782/upj/2023-1-6

Ellman, S. J. (1997). Criteria for termination. *Psychoanalytic Psychology*, 14(2), 197–210. https://doi.org/10.1037/h0079716

Freud, S. (1914). On narcissism: An introduction. *Standard Edition*, 14, 73–102.

Freud, S. (1959). Analysis terminable and interminable. *The Psychoanalytic Review*, 26, 237.

Gabbard, G. O. (2009). What is a "good enough" termination? *Journal of the American Psychoanalytic Association*, 57(3), 575–594. https://doi.org/10.1177/0003065109340678

Green, A. (2018). *Resonance of suffering: Countertransference in non-neurotic structures*. Routledge.

Grenell, G. (2002). The termination phase of psychoanalysis as seen through the lens of the dream. *Journal of the American Psychoanalytic Association*, 50(3), 779–805. https://doi.org/10.1177/00030651020500030901

Grossmark, R. (2020). It's all too much: Excess, enactment and ending in Danielle Knafo's "The sexual illusionist." *Psychoanalytic Perspectives*, 17(1), 41–52. https://doi.org/10.1080/1551806X.2019.1685310

Holmes, J. (2011). Termination in psychoanalytic psychotherapy: An attachment perspective. In J. Salberg (Ed.) *Good enough endings* (pp. 87–106). Routledge.

Kantrowitz, J. L. (2014). *Myths of termination: What patients can teach psychoanalysts about endings*. Routledge.

Knafo, D. (2018). Beginnings and endings: Time and termination in psychoanalysis. *Psychoanalytic Psychology*, 35(1), 8. http://dx.doi.org/10.1037/pap0000125

Lagutin, V. (2023). Psychoanalysis "traumatized" by war. Four clinical illustrations of the vulnerability of the setting. *Ukrainian Psychoanalytic Journal*, 1(3), 18–23. https://doi.org/10.32782/upj/2023-3-3

Lazos, G. (2023). Transformation of psychotherapeutic relationships during the war. *Psychoanalysis, Self and Context*, 18(3), 382–387. https://doi.org/10.1080/24720038.2023.2203158

Lussana, S. (2018). Termination of a psychoanalysis: Some notes on theory, technique, and clinical material. *The International Journal of Psychoanalysis*, 99(3), 603–626. https://doi.org/10.1080/00207578.2017.1399067

Nalyvaiko, N. (2023). Borders and psychoanalysis in a time of war. *Psychoanalytic Psychology*, 40(4). http://doi.org/10.1037/pap0000485

Orgel, S. (2000). Letting go: Some thoughts about termination. *Journal of the American Psychoanalytic Association*, 48(3), 719–738. https://doi.org/10.1177/00030651000480031601

Pediconi, M. G. (2019). Beyond termination Freud and Lacan on healing: Principles and practice. *DIVISION*. https://societaamicidelpensiero.it/wp-content/uploads/GP_atlanta_Beyond_Termination.pdf

Power, A. (2015). *Forced endings in psychotherapy and psychoanalysis: Attachment and loss in retirement*. Routledge.

Romanov, I. (2023). The war inside: Unconscious experience of war in a patient and an analyst. *KnotGarden*, 2, 67–85.

Salberg, J. (2014). Leaning into termination: Finding a good-enough ending. In *Relational psychoanalysis* (Vol. 5, pp. 331–351). Routledge.

Schlesinger, H. (2013). *Endings and beginnings: On terminating psychotherapy and psychoanalysis*. Routledge.

Shane, E. (2009). Approaching termination: Ideal criteria versus working realities. *Psychoanalytic Inquiry*, 29(2), 167–173. https://doi.org/10.1080/07351690802274876

Skolnick, N. J. (2011). Termination in psychoanalysis: It's about time. In J. Salberg (Ed.) *Good enough endings* (pp. 247–264). Routledge.

Velykodna, M. (2023). A psychoanalyst's experience of working in wartime: On choosing between bad options. *Psychoanalytic Psychology*, 40(4). http://doi.org/10.1037/pap0000480

Winnicott, D. W. (2018). Transitional objects and transitional phenomena 1—a study of the first not-me possession 2. In A. C. Furman, and S. T. Levy (Eds.), *Influential papers from the 1950s* (pp. 202–221). Routledge.

Zimmer, R. (2021). Post-termination self-analysis and the relinquishment of the psychoanalytic frame: Thoughts on a fragment of self-analytic work following a traumatic termination. *The International Journal of Psychoanalysis*, 102(6), 1116–1137. https://doi.org/10.1080/00207578.2021.1904780

Chapter 9

Avoiding Talking about the War? Features of Transference During Counseling with Ukrainian Refugees

Elina Yevlanova

East or west, home is best.

(English proverb)

In February 2022, after the invasion of Russian troops into Ukraine, my family and I found ourselves among millions of Ukrainians who left their homes in search of safe cities to survive. To a large extent, my family was lucky: we found shelter in the Ukrainian city where I spent my childhood, where my oldest child was born, where my parents are buried, and where my relatives and friends still live. This city is located in the central part of Ukraine, which was also hit by Russian rockets, but my family and I felt much safer than in Kyiv in the first months of the war. Thus, we did not have to face those days full of despair and unspeakable horror, facing numerous refugee problems that I learned about and continue to learn about during analysis with my patients. In May 2022, my family and I returned to our home in Kyiv, which fortunately remained intact. Many Ukrainian families could not return to their homes.

According to the official data on September 30, 2023, the number of Ukrainian refugees in the European Union countries alone was more than 4 million people, and there were nearly 7 million Ukrainian refugees worldwide (UNHCR – The UN Refugee Agency). Moreover, Ukraine has two types of groups considered displaced: refugees who moved across the borders and internally displaced persons who were forcibly moved to other cities and villages in Ukraine. Almost twice as many Ukrainians are considered internally displaced as refugees. Thus, an enormous number of Ukrainians (from a population of about 40 million) have been forcibly displaced from their homes, fleeing to safety in other areas of the country or the world.

DOI: 10.4324/9781032660257-10

Therefore, the psychoanalytic practice shifted to working with numerous individuals who live away from their homes, whether in other cities of Ukraine or other countries. In this article, I explore the phenomena I encountered while working with Ukrainian refugees and internally displaced persons. Within a month of Russia's full-scale invasion, as a psychoanalyst, I began listening to stories my patients shared with me about their lives, which were drastically changed by conditions outside of their control. These stories varied, depending on many factors. Among my patients are many women of all ages who fled abroad with their children, as well as many young Ukrainian teens and young adults who either fled together with their parents or with only their friends. Some of these patients return to Ukraine from time to time; others do not because of significant fear, yet others decide to return permanently to Ukraine and live in their own homes. Among my patients who still live in a foreign country as refugees, the adaptation processes are markedly different. First, this difference is accounted for by the individual patterns of their mental functioning. In addition, these differences are shaped by such factors as people's ability to learn the language of a host country, their intentions of returning to Ukraine in the future, and their opportunities to engage in their established professional activities. For example, patients who can maintain work in their chosen career or have access to continuing their education online have different adaptation patterns than those individuals who are forced to take up employment outside of their career background, often in the low-skilled job sector. Moreover, individuals who can maintain relative career stability appear to be more capable of learning the new language as well as becoming more open to exploring new relationships or their host location.

Finally, as I discussed below, as psychoanalysts, we are trained to analyze patients' unconscious material by paying special attention to their language or patterns of speech. In our training, we are invited to recognize and work with unconscious dynamics, specifically through what and how patients say about their internal and external lives. In this chapter, I describe a different experience of working with the unconscious. Based on the classic works of Sigmund Freud, Jacques Lacan, Francoise Dolto, and others, I examine the phenomenon of patients actively "not talking" about the war, which is especially common with patients who experienced direct life-threatening war violence and danger as they fled their homes and their country.

When "Cozy" Becomes "Uncanny"

In the first days of the war, millions of Ukrainians faced the reality that their houses and apartments were no longer safe. To save their own lives and the lives of their children, they had to flee to other areas. In my and our Ukrainian experience, this war revealed how helpless modern human beings are in the face of catastrophes and how deceptive are our ideas about the protections offered by the walls of our homes. "My home is my castle" loses all meaning. And then, despite homes of return to home and safety, many people are forced to remain displaced as the war machine continues to bring endless forms of violence.

Thus, my practice became oriented toward working with Ukrainians, many of whom remained refugees across the borders now for over two years. Most of my patients are currently residing in various European countries, as well as in the United States. Some of them hoped to return to Ukraine, whereas others embraced the fact that they might be unable to return and have to settle in countries that offered them shelter. Their stories are very different, just as their mental capacities and psychic dynamics. However, in the stories of my refugee patients, one feature remains constant: most of them rarely, if ever, talk about the war in Ukraine in our sessions. At the beginning of the war, I attributed this pattern to the fact that refugees, especially adults, were facing an enormous amount of stressful life pressure to adapt to their lives in another country. Perhaps, I surmised, they had enough mental resources to feel safe in the "here and now." Yet, as months passed, and as we shifted from crisis or supportive therapy back to psychoanalytic work, the topic of war remained as if it were a taboo. Words about the war typically did not enter our therapeutic space. In his *Roman Discourse,* Jacques Lacan (1955) stressed that whatever psychoanalysis seeks to achieve, be it healing, professional training, or research, its medium is rooted in the patient's speech. Psychoanalysts are trained to approach patient's words with the hope of finding the material that is being silenced. Then what if the most glaring of life conditions is never named in words?

Thus, a question emerged for me: "Why are my patients silent about the war?" and I brought it into my clinical supervision. I recognized that in the transference space, I brought in my reality as having been an "internally displaced person." I, too, vividly recall having to flee my home. I remember the fear that there might not be time to escape: no time to leave the building because a missile might hit it, or not having time to escape by car because it might be bombed or shot at by the Russian soldiers, and then not having time to drive past the area, where the Russian tanks were about to appear. Fortunately for me, my family and I managed to pass these dangerous parts, but barely two hours before the Russian tanks invaded the territory. These tanks proceeded to fire at civilian cars and structures, and as shown in massacres in Bucha and elsewhere, were used to commit numerous atrocities (e.g., rolling over burnt bodies of tortured Ukrainians). I certainly remembered those stressful hours well, so maybe in the transference space, I was not ready to revisit those memories again and again through the experiences of my patients, thus unconsciously communicating with them my reluctance to discuss the war. My supervision helped me to identify and acknowledge my countertransferential resistance to discussing the topic of war.

However, after bringing greater awareness to these transferential possibilities, I still found myself puzzled by both the absence of material about the war in my patients' stories as well as my confusion about whether and how to bring this up with them. It became clear to me with time that if I pretended that the war did not exist, I could be colluding with my patients' symptoms. The consequence of acknowledging this defensive modality and resistance, I worried, may disrupt the space of psychoanalytic treatment by bringing war into it. Specifically, inquiring about the war with my patients could be perceived as counter-transference, acting out rather than holding my analytic stance via interpretation. It could become an interruption of the analysis and the analytic goals brought in by the patients. I held many doubts and worries while also realizing that this ever-present absence of talking about the war was intersubjectively charged in our treatments.

After these deliberations and observations, I decided to refer to the theme of the war in my words to my patients, or rather, I highlighted their absence as a metaphor. In Lacan's (1955) words, a "synonym of the symptom of symbolic displacement included in the mechanism" must be framed via the speech as an ellipse. In literature, an ellipsis is a stylistic choice that denotes an omission of a certain part of a sentence or a phrase (i.e., to achieve dynamism and tension of the action he describes, the author omits some structural elements of the sentence that can be easily guessed by the reader based on the context or content of the poetic speech). In psychoanalytic practice, ellipses, like circumlocutions, can be viewed as possibilities for the unconscious to emerge. I had a fantasy of my patients writing their life stories but seeking to omit an entire chapter.

Thus, I began to perceive their silence as a censored chapter, but I also began to recognize that it had been recorded somewhere else within the psychic space in patients' minds.

In his work entitled *On Aphasia*, Freud (Davison, 1955; Freud & Strachey, 2001) examined the nature of the aphasic disorder from a psychological point of view. Notably, the word "aphasia" is derived from the Greek "aphasis" which translates as being "without speech." In this work, Freud differentiated aphasia (i.e., partial or complete loss of speech) as the result of a focal lesion of the brain in contrast to psychological speech disorders, which he observed among his patients with hysteria. Freud noted that in patients with hysteria, speech reflected verbal and objective representations found in the psyche, and he examined the connection between the occurrences of speech of any length among such patients and the images embedded in their words. He considered verbal representation as a closed complex (i.e., sounds, letters, utterances), while words with object representation were viewed as an open defensive pattern. In his later works, Freud (1936) further developed this theory toward recognition of unconscious mnemonic images. These images could be used to make up a catalog of what a person perceives, remembers, and traces of their individual experience. Words and speech, in Freud's view, held capacities to stimulate libidinal excitement. His further establishing key psychoanalytic concepts revealed that speech and directly articulating words are the primary ways to make unconscious material conscious, thus placing the unconscious under the control of Ego. Thus, speaking words about images and patterns is central to the psychoanalytic process of working with the unconscious.

Another aspect of language in this war is related to Russia's insistence on erasing the Ukrainian language. I recollect one of our first group therapy sessions, meeting the day after the invasion and then a month later. Within a month, all of the group members had to flee their homes. What was striking was that all of them switched to speaking in Ukrainian, even though before the invasion, the majority of the group members were still predominately Russian speaking (i.e., for many centuries, Ukraine was first a part of the Russian Empire and then of the Soviet Union with an emphasis on linguistic control from Moscow). One of the rules of the group, which I announced at our first meeting long before the war began, stressed that everyone was free to speak the language they were comfortable with, and the group operated as bilingual (both Ukrainian and Russian). Yet, in our first meetings following the invasion, I noted to the group that everyone purposefully switched to the Ukrainian language with no prompting. The choice of language by group members denoted that the Russian language reflected Russian aggression, evoking tremendous affective reactions. In addition, everyone in the group had to abandon their homes because they were also marked for destruction by the Russian aggressor, evoking similarly powerful affects. Thus, in our shared group metaphor, the Ukrainian language became a symbol of home and security, which were being preserved via newly constructed relation to the Ukrainian language. For months and months, we met every week.

As I write these lines, it is difficult to convey my feelings in those days: every meeting with every patient, I held the thought that either they or I could be killed in a Russian strike. Every one of my colleagues and group members faced similar threats every moment of every day (and many still do). Every dynamic in the therapy group I led remains with me. I recall that one of the group members shared that she was pregnant with her first child, but other than hearing this from a physician and sharing it with her husband, no one was left to share her news with.

Notably, therapeutic space can, at times, become challenging or dangerous when splits in the patient's psyche are activated in the process of work, and the analyst (i.e., analytic group, office, online space) is experienced as posing a threat to the patient's existence. These occurrences are understood as negative transference, which may be caused by regressive experiences of difficult early relationships. However, since the beginning of the war, Ukrainian patients and analysts found themselves in real situations of threat of destruction and persecution by the enemy who attacked their homes. Therapy emerges as a space for patients to experience whatever arises in their psychic and external lives in such times. I have also come to believe that it is essential that the analyst can manage such regressive states under conditions of actual threat to life.

For most human beings, the home represents the internal capacity to experience safety and happiness. During the war, as the home is threatened, people can also react differently to perceive threats based on the structure of their mental defenses. Many Ukrainians I work with, recalling the first days of the war, focus on their efforts to calm themselves with various "rational" thoughts. For many Ukrainians, rationalizations included "this can't be a real war," "maybe Russians are using bombings and force to try to negotiate," "Russia would never attack Kyiv," "they aren't really trying to occupy Ukraine," or "they are just trying to use temporary scare tactics." These rationalizations certainly reflect attempts to reduce extreme states of anxiety in the face of war. However, within the first few days of the invasion, all such "rational" thoughts were dispelled with the reality, and Ukrainians began to flee away from active war zones and the borders with Russia.

"The war arrived at my home's door" – many cultures use this expression in more metaphoric ways. This phrase typically denotes personal life and boundaries, but for many in Ukraine and worldwide, it certainly carries the meaning of attacks on one's country, community, and actual home. Regardless of the context, this turn of phrase always denotes something negative – an invasion of one's psychic and external life. For many Ukrainians, thoughts of "home" immediately evoke images of horror with signifiers such as the "Russian language," "East," "occupier," "war," and "enemy." In etymological terms, the Romance language use of the words "home" and "house" is derived from the Proto-Germanic sources – old English "hām," of Germanic origin; related to Dutch "heem" and German "Heim." Old English terms for a house are "hūs" (noun), and "hūsian" (verb), of Germanic origin and are also related to Dutch "huis," German "Haus" (nouns), and Dutch "huizen," and German "hausen" (verbs). I wished to include these Romance and Germanic words to turn the attention to ways, in which Freud (1976) used them creatively in his work *The Uncanny*. He used them throughout his essay in varied forms of opposition between German words for "known, comfortable" and "secret, that which is hidden from the eyes of a stranger." Freud's writing engages the concept of semantic unity in his Heimlich – Unheimlich, which he uses to differentiate between what is the internal and the external. In his writing, these words focus on the concept of negation and on "something that should always remain ambivalent." In clinical illustrations presented below, I further discuss the challenges of working with Ukrainian refugees for whom the linguistic psychic capacity to name the war is just as psychically impossible as naming varied aspects of their home in the world.

Clinical Illustration One

Patient M is a 20-year-old student at one of the Kyiv universities. She grew up with her parents and older sister, who appeared to have been generally supportive and caring for M throughout her life. When we began our work in May of 2023, she temporarily lived in the Czech Republic with her sister, who was already living there before the war. The patient's primary concerns were her social anxiety and her incapacity to manage stress. During the intake, I learned that M's "social anxiety" was manifest in her incapacity to leave the house on her own. This pattern caused quarrels with her sister, who told M that she was merely being difficult and lazy. Their parents remained living in Kyiv but were able to visit their daughters from time to time during the war. Her parents tried to get her out of the house with varied invitations for sightseeing, but M typically found ways to refuse, which was met with further family arguments. During our sessions, M mostly discussed her college studies, although she also shared about the lack of acceptance of Ukrainians by the host community, about arguments with her parents, and, occasionally, about her interactions with her fellow students. M's life goals seemed to be focused on achieving top grades in her college classes with the explicit goal of obtaining a well-paying job following her education. M showed no interest in romantic relationships and, using Freud's (Breuer & Freud, 2009) similar observation of his patient, "didn't want to know anything about sexual relationships." In our sessions, I experienced her as gifted intellectually, engaging, and attractive but as radiating enormous anxiety and fear, which she often sought to disguise with intellectual rationalizations. For instance, one of her resistance strategies appeared as her "inability" to make associations: her communication often felt as if she was looking for test questions, which she answered in a "correct" manner. This form of control over the analytic process appeared as her defensive strategy for avoiding her anxiety, resisting any doubt, and refusing uncertainty. At times when her defenses were lowered, M could let me see that she was a sensitive, deeply caring, and timid person.

M's defenses and her anxiety are best understood in the context of her life through Russia's war against Ukraine. Until 2014, M and her family lived in the city of Donetsk, which was occupied in 2014 and remains under Russian occupation. Her family lived in their own house and her parents held good jobs. She describes her growing up as very social, spending time with many friends and numerous relatives. When the war arrived in Eastern Ukraine, M's parents sent her, her sister, and a grandmother to Turkey. At that time, the family hoped that within a month or two, the hostilities would be over, and their lives would return to normality they had known before the war. But within a month of Russia's war, it became clear to them that the city was now occupied, and the war persisted. M's parents moved to Kyiv, managing to keep their jobs, while M's older sister went abroad to study at a university. Thus, at age 11, faced with enormous war losses, M fled her home and her home life, ending up in Kyiv. M shared that through this change, she felt relatively stable and that she was able to make many new friends and succeed in her new school environment. Nevertheless, she also shared that this transition, at times, was difficult and fraught and that she also felt like a "stranger" in this new place. Because so-called para-military "separatists" from the Donbas area of Ukraine aligned themselves with the Russian military, many Ukrainians did not fully trust people like her family from Eastern Ukraine; she shared that Kyiv never fully became a new home for her. And then, in the winter of 2022, she found herself displaced and losing her home once again, fleeing to be with her sister across the border. Again, the war was uncertain and indeterminable, and again, she was a person with limited rights.

Her symptoms of social anxiety appeared to decrease after she visited Ukraine and her parents in the summer of 2023, reporting that she could take some impromptu walks outside her home. But M continued to report that being in any crowded space (e.g., supermarket) was extremely anxiety-provoking for her, stating that she felt like a "hostage." She shared that she continued to prefer remaining at home as much as she could but that she was far more distressed about her inability to manage her anxiety and leave the confines of her house. Notably, her symptoms are striking defensive forms of psychic adaptation, which kept her "hostage" in her own home but also become a form of identification with an aggressor because it was she who kept herself in this "hostage" situation. As Freud (1917, 2014) aptly showed, each neurotic symptom points to the duality of psychic defensive mechanisms. Moreover, M certainly experienced numerous encounters with actual military and war hostage situations: at one point in our work, she recalled being held at gunpoint by a Russian "separatist." M also recalled with time that, possibly precipitated by war violence and escaping Donetsk, her menstrual cycle began at age 11, right as the family was fleeing their home. Her family home in Donetsk was not taken over and occupied by a Russian family, but millions of Russians en-mass descended on occupied areas of Crimea and Eastern Ukraine after Russian occupation and stole homes, possessions, businesses, and all other Ukrainians' property. The violent occupiers occupying her childhood town also occupied M's imagination. Her child's psyche was burdened by developing war just as her own body was developing toward its next stage. Moreover, the oedipal complications M faced in her developmental because of what happened to her family of origin also shaped her psychic life. External sadism became what M had to face, but also psychically integrate, which over time led to the intense rejection of all social relations and contacts. In addition, her somatic "home" experienced and held many forms of expulsion and aggressive exclusion, which is also reflected in her unconscious communications of what it means to "leave home."

As Dolto (Dolto & Bailly, 2022) highlighted, early unprocessed forms of severe trauma can damage the capacity to symbolize and metabolize when faced with new trauma as adults.

War is violence. In my view, psychoanalysts must pay close attention to what patients share in analytic settings to tease out the phantasies and psychic experiences based on early (unconsciously held) histories from ongoing trauma of war. In many ways, I believe such distinction is, at times, nearly impossible to make because patients with such histories tend to weave their past horrors together with present-day ones. What helps me work in situations of this increased uncertainty is the ethics of the psychoanalytic process because psychoanalytic space can become a container for new ways of knowing, it can become a space where the acknowledgment of resistance to knowing is permitted, a space for understanding of psychic defenses and phantasies, but also the space where we as analysts can openly renounce the illusory power that patients unconsciously grant us in the transference phenomenon (i.e., mutually accept not knowing). Thus, in the conditions of war, trying to be "opaque to the subject, and like a mirror to show nothing but what is shown to him" (Freud, 2014) is not always within the therapist's power to grant. Moreover, from my own experience, in many cases, my greater openness in the sessions (especially at the beginning of the war) had a profoundly salubrious therapeutic effect. However, I have also come to understand that every moment of "transparency" by me as an analyst also enters enactments and transferential space. I believe, therefore, it is important to return to all disclosures or breaks in the therapeutic frame in the following sessions.

During the war, the pull to relieve the patient's suffering or to name symptoms to control them became significant. However, even in such conditions, I have found that it is important that regardless of our pull to help, our psycho-educational interventions, or symptom management technique, we must recognize that these cannot substitute the difficult work with challenging psychic material. As Freud (1936) aptly suggested, helping the patient to alleviate conditions by direct intervention functions in the same way as reading the menu in a restaurant can help a hungry person.

Anxiety as Avoidance of Facing the War

Theory about the inhibition-symptom-anxiety triad, defined by Freud (1936) in the work of the same name and further developed by Jacques Lacan (2011) in his "Anxiety" seminar, stresses that psychic energy is often directed at the avoidance of experiencing anxiety. Moreover, defensive inhibitions and symptoms are often psychic "constructions" that facilitate this avoidance. Certainly, for a person who was forced to leave home to flee occupation, shelling, or rocket attacks, the state of anxiety is caused by fear for one's own life and the uncertainty of the future in a foreign land. However, what I observed in clinical practice is that a large number of patients seek psychotherapy for varied forms of generalized anxiety while acting paralyzed when faced with making life decisions, such as about employment, therefore undermining their adaptation. Understandably, their anxiety is undoubtedly a manifestation of actual trauma as well as their developmental trauma or challenges when regression prevents the person from engaging productively with their lives. In a typical process of analysis with such patients, we often begin with supportive interpretations, usually focused on containing the patient's anxiety. However, during times of war, I have found that interpretations related to patients' history and their transference reactions should be avoided, giving preference to the interpretations of their present experiences (and current events) and the interpretations outside of transference (Etchegoyen, 2018). During this period of work, it is important to maintain the "controlled regression" (Winnicott, 2016), remembering that at some point patient's anxiety level may become unbearable (Lacan, 2011), that the patient is ready to move through their anxiety toward working through can be found in a new signifier, which can symbolize the transition of the patient's psyche from living within the dimension of demands to a dimension of desire. I have termed this moment in therapy as the moment of the symbolic birth of the "refugee," which in my clinical experience typically appears with a word or words that are associated with strong affects (i.e., shame and guilt for one's helplessness) rather than anxiety. Some of my Ukrainian patients seem to pass into this stage within a few months of their relocation, while others may be "stuck" in their anxiety for 12–16 months. The following case illustration highlights my theoretical and clinical observations.

Clinical Illustration Two

Patient V is an 18-year-old psychology student at one of Kyiv's universities. At the beginning of the war, he, along with his mother and younger brother, fled Kyiv to Romania, where they lived for several months. At that time, his mother and brother returned to Kyiv, where his father and grandparents stayed behind, while V moved to Portugal, where he lived with his girlfriend and her family. At the time of our assessment, V appeared extremely agitated. He complained of sleep disturbance, anxiety, and panic attacks. It was difficult for him to name the exact date of his birth or recall the timing of his arrival in Portugal. He often was confused about the time of our appointments and would end up initiating sessions not from the privacy of his apartment but from a park. He believed that his difficult anxiety condition was related to his use of mild marijuana he smoked while in Romania. He emphasized that his smoking led to his panic attacks and was insistent on avoiding all drugs other than vaping. During our initial session, he was filled with severe anxiety about being apprehended by the Portuguese police for his supposed "drug offenses" in Romania, even though he consumed a very small amount and was not involved in distribution. He also seemed to interpret any interaction with neighbors or his landlord as either aggressive or as laughing at him. V was exhausted from insomnia as well as continually feeling agitated and irritable. During the early stages of treatment, he perceived me transferentially as his mother (his mother was, in fact, a psychologist). He tried, in his words, to be "the omniscient son of an omniscient mother." When he did not talk about his persecutory fears or perceived hostility toward him, he often turned to highly intellectual topics he was learning in his psychology program, such as psychogenetics. During episodes of severe anxiety, he also sought to find the source of his anxiety in phantasies about having an incurable illness or about the sudden death of his girlfriend. I observed that an early paranoid part of his Ego often alternated with the more mature defense of intellectualization when some connection to reality prevailed. Like many psychotically organized patients, he seemed to search for answers about himself while contending with an image of a mother who is libidinally powerful and omnipotent (Brunswick, 1940).

He first spoke about the war when he returned to Kyiv in the summer of 2023 (a year and a half after the day of the invasion). The topic came up when V missed his session due to an air raid: he and his friends had to hide from a rocket attack in one of the subway stations. This became an important moment in therapy. It should be noted that the Ukrainian word "[tryvoha]" is used both about external warning sound that warns of danger (alarm) as well as a mental phenomenon of agitation (anxiety). This experience and the words about the war that emerged in our work became central to working through his anxiety.

First, his anxiety seemed to have acquired a real object in the external real world – the Russian missiles. Second, V's anxiety acquired another Oedipal dimension, in which a third appeared – a mythical all-powerful "father" who wanted to harm him. This image for V included both Putin, who sought to destroy V for being Ukrainian, but also in his worry about the Ukrainian authorities, which could demand that he go to the frontlines, albeit the laws in Ukraine permitted enrolled university students to refuse mobilization. Thus, the public Big Other (Lacan, 1955) – the Ukrainian government became for V both a figure of threat but also of protection, who wanted V to learn and to live.

In our subsequent sessions, I began to see an ordinary teenager in front of me. He seemed to be saying goodbye to his childhood memories and, at the same time, constructing himself in a new, unconscious world. His stories were now full of memories of his father, who once helped him overcome his childhood fears. In our sessions, he often talked of men in his memories and his life: in addition to his father, it was his brother, uncle, grandfather, and friends. When he initiated termination, he still reported having anxious thoughts and doubts, but he seemed to have far more capacity to engage with his life and his symptoms without resorting to anxiety. Moreover, when V left his native home in Kyiv, he became a person who did not just lose his home but also his memories and his past. Working through anxiety via symbolization and mentalization of actual war experiences and words, he once again located himself within a symbolic system of his family and lineage. The adolescent period, which is characterized by the reactivation of Oedipal experiences (Freud & Strachey, 2001), for V, occurred at the time of war and exile when being a man and a Ukrainian man became dangerous. Moreover, since the majority of Ukrainian refugees are women and children, he also could not locate himself within a symbolic community of displaced people.

A Loss That Cannot Be Named

The word "refugee" in English, according to dictionaries, appeared in usage during the early 17th century (originally referring to Protestants who fled France to seek "refuge" from religious persecution in other areas). In the French language, the word also denotes someone or something that is "gone." The Ukrainian word for refugee – [bizhenets] – uses an imagery of a person who runs or escapes (i.e., [bizhyt]). The Ukrainian word has a direction – running "from something." Until 2014 and in the following years, Ukraine itself hosted many refugees – usually people who escaped totalitarianism and political violence, including from Russia and Belarus. In addition, refugees (including in media images) are people who are desperate, poor, and devastated. Until 2014, most Ukrainians could not perceive themselves in such conditions since most Ukrainians enjoyed a fairly high standard of living. In 2014, waves of millions of Ukrainian refugees from the East of Ukraine and Crimea streamed in to find shelter and establish new lives albeit most of them remained internally in Ukraine. After the invasion of 2022, it is estimated that almost one in two Ukrainians became refugees, millions fleeing with nothing across the borders. Facing life as a refugee in a foreign country is often marked not only by direct war trauma but by narcissistic injury to healthy human capacities to be able to control and direct their lives. Discussions of war for many refugees are extremely challenging since these painful internal realities are activated. When I asked one woman I ended up a refugee in Great Britain about whether she discussed war with her Ukrainian friends, she responded: "We didn't escape the war to talk about it." In truth, I understand her efforts not to speak, not to think, not to encounter mental pain, or not to face grief, guilt, and other emotions (Steiner, 2022). In the following case, a patient refuses to discuss war in our treatment for almost 20 months of our work.

Clinical Illustration Three

Before the war, patient N attended a support group for people whose relatives have dementia, which I facilitated because her father had Alzheimer's disease. As I mentioned earlier, I continued the work with groups even after the full-scale invasion. N attended our group from France, where she ended up as a refugee with her children. When N's father died, N began to skip the group or, when she participated, appeared unemotional, robotic, and numb. As an analyst, looking back, I now wonder if I engaged too precipitously in offering N to begin individual analysis with me. In addition to agreeing that she would drop out of the group and begin individual sessions, I was also moved by her financial situation and her loss of her job, offering her my services for free. Looking back, I know that during the first weeks and months of war offering analytic services for free served to combat my helplessness in the face of unbearable war but also reflected my belief that the war could only end quickly (how can such inhumane conditions be permitted to exist or to last?).

During initial individual sessions, N repeatedly complained about the feeling as if a granite slab was placed on her chest, which inhibited her from feeling or crying. In our sessions, N processed not only her father's death but also the fact that because her father was moved for safety to Poland and died there, N had to navigate processes and documents related to death and burial in a foreign country with no knowledge of its language or customs. While it appeared that Polish authorities were very helpful, she seemed to feel complicated grief and confusion about her decisions. Our sessions switched between her problems in France (e.g., helplessness, overwhelm) and issues with bringing her father's ashes back to Ukraine, yet in the midst of it, N continually omitted key significant aspects of her life. In our sessions, N seemed intellectually capable but highly controlled and educative in her presentation. In transference, I felt that she treated me as a parent with dementia as well as someone who was merely a mirror for her to reflect her correct ways of speaking or acting. In fact, at one time, she kindly said to me during a session, "You must have forgotten what I told you, but it's OK. I'll tell you again." I recall that at that time, she cried and showed more affect in speaking to me, but I was aware that after months and months of analysis, she seemed unable to make any associations to her symptoms.

In classic analytic work, formulation of a symptom is a key part of accessing the unconscious processes, including by paying attention to its manifestation in the analysis itself. In everyday life, a symptom in its essence is when something hinders individuals and is perceived as an obstacle. In the analytical space, varied forms of symptomatic repetition are typically present and analyzed. First is the symptom itself. In the case of a hysterical patient, it is a conversion symptom. Second, the symptom is viewed as playing out an internal conflict outside of analytical sessions. Third, symptoms are a form of acting out (Lacan, 2011). In working with N, I wondered what the symptom is, how it is manifested in our work and her life, and whether or not I was engaged in countertransferential enactments with N, which did not let me have access to it.

In a session in the summer of 2022, half a year after the invasion, N joined our session from the train station in France. She was sobbing, unable to speak, saying she was lost, that she missed her train and did not know how to get home. She demonstrated a lack of orientation to space and place. I asked her to find a safe place and insisted we continue our session. In contrast to our typical sessions from her temporary home, in this session, after calming down, N was finally able to name her profound loneliness as well as her struggles with living in a foreign country, both morally and materially. What also emerged after this experience was our return to discussing payment for our sessions because continuing to work for free also created a conflict both with her and between us. When I asked her how she felt about renewing our financial commitments, N responded: "Money is a relationship." She seemed connected to me in ways that she has not been in other sessions. This experience reminded me of the importance of payment as part of the therapeutic frame, which Freud discussed, but also recognition that her financial arrangement with me maintained her capacity to remain in a professional relationship as a Ukrainian with me as a Ukrainian, even while a refugee. Her narcissistic injury about being destitute seemed also to be helped by establishing a doable payment schedule.

In addition to working through this aspect of our enactment, I also began to recognize that N was identified with the dementia of her deceased father, for whom she cared in Ukraine and whose loss was mired in her refugee experience. She developed a kind of inner dementia toward her mind and experiences, which served as an identification with her father. When a person experiences the loss of a loved one, and when object relations become impossible or complicated, challenging object identifications can degrade into symptoms – melancholia rather than mourning (Freud, 1917).

Notably, with time, money and payment for treatment became the object of the reality of our analytic relationship, which seemed to affirm to her both my existence and her existence, helping to move from narcissistic injury toward object libidinal relations (Freud, 2014). Our session in the train station also marked the beginning of her grieving work. In her history, N experienced other deaths, which she managed by prohibiting herself from thinking or feeling. She also refused to think about the war or her husband, relatives, and friends in Ukraine, seemingly in a defensive form of denial and omnipotence – "If I don't think about it, nothing bad will happen." To recognize herself as an unemployed refugee, as being now poor and an orphan became signifiers, which N resisted when she kept silent about the war during our sessions. The anxiety that gripped her at the train station was also related to feelings of shame, which she tried to avoid – in his work entitled The *Roman Discourse,* Lacan (1955) related Freud's initial claim, also stating that the symptom is always overdetermined. With greater emphasis on language and words as forms of free association, Lacan emphasized that in the intersections of verbal forms and their analysis, the "symptom is completely refuted, because it is structured as a language; that he, in other words, is the language whose speech must be liberated" in the process of psychoanalytic treatment. For N, these were words about limits, mortality, guilt, and death.

Conclusion

Refugees are a direct symptom and a long-term consequence of wars. It is precisely because of the refugees that the war, without exaggeration, becomes visible and tangible far beyond the geographical boundaries of the territory on which militarized violence is unleashed. The situation in which people try to escape immediate danger to their lives by fleeing their own homes and seeking safety in other countries has always been extremely traumatic for human mental health and the subsequent adaptation of refugees. These significant challenges also follow the next generations of their descendants.

When I realized that my refugee patients avoided talking about the war in our sessions, I thought not only about them but also their children. I imagined that these children will face the future in which they, too, are taught to avoid thinking or talking about what impacts their lives, at times in unbearably difficult ways. I realized that if I took up the directives from classic analytic techniques and followed my analysts while waiting for the speech to emerge, I would make a mistake. Moreover, I now also believe that my resistance to discussing war directly was part of my avoidance of talking about profoundly difficult things in my own life. After facing my resistance to talking about the war, I was able to treat my patients' "not talking about the war" as a symptom, not a symptom to "treat," but to analytically investigate. My work revealed the enormous amount of mental stress that war and displacement brought to a person's mental life. This tension could not be processed by their normal mental structures, and therefore, their psychic required help in processing this material.

For the refugee to emerge in our treatment, the patient had to speak about the war, and I, as a psychoanalyst, had to be ready to return, again and again, to the memories of morning explosions in February 2022, when I fled my home and faced unbearable confusion and helplessness. These events from my life mirror precisely the stories of each of my refugee patients. While I had to bear, time and again, the memories of horror, this process was essential in helping me understand what my patients were going through in our sessions.

When the dynamics in our therapeutic work shifted as words for the "unspeakable" were found, I finally seemed to be able to accept how indescribable the horrors of war are for human beings. From now on, I will include war in the list of primary topics that are brought into initial sessions with all of my new Ukrainian patients. I certainly am not suggesting that analysts ask "Tell me about the war" within a list of biographical intake questions about age, family, or occupation. Yet open introduction and permission to discuss the war will be included with all of them. Every time I ask, "Do you remember how you felt when you realized the war had started?" I try to choose a moment when this question can play the role of interpreting the patient's stories.

Certainly, I recognize that in such cases, as in all of our work, the analyst must be prepared for the patient's strong transference reaction, as well as strong countertransference feelings. Yet, in the acknowledgment of war, the analyst also invites the patients to understand that the analyst can withstand the onslaught of enormously strong feelings and memories while remaining whole. This condition becomes essential in establishing therapeutic relationships with Ukrainian refugees (and all Ukrainian patients). The patients then recognize that their experience in therapy can include stories about the unspeakable and that they can be with this experience together with the therapist. Perhaps this experience is also about building a safe container in the initial sessions, in which the patient can talk about the war as a prerequisite for our shared capacity to withstand the anxiety of the analytic process.

References

Breuer, J., & Freud, S. (2009). *Studies on hysteria*. Hachette.

Brunswick, R. M. (1940). The preoedipal phase of the libido development. *The Psychoanalytic Quarterly*, 9(2), 293–319.

Davison, C. (1955). On aphasia (A critical study). By S. Freud. Translated by E. Stengel. International Universities Press, Inc., 1953. 105 pp.

Dolto, F., & Bailly, S. (2022). The unconscious body image. In Baiily (Ed.) *The unconscious body image* (pp. 8–44). Routledge.

Etchegoyen, R. H. (2018). *The fundamentals of psychoanalytic technique*. Routledge.

Freud, S. (1917). Mourning and melancholia. In *The standard edition of the complete psychological works of Sigmund Freud, Volume XIV (1914–1916): On the history of the psycho-analytic movement, papers on metapsychology and other Works* (pp. 237–258). London: Hogarth Press

Freud, S. (1936). Inhibitions, symptoms, and anxiety. *The Psychoanalytic Quarterly*, 5(1), 1–28.

Freud, S. (1976). The uncanny. *New Literary History*, 7(3), 525–645.

Freud, S. (2014). *On narcissism: An introduction*. Read Books Ltd.

Freud, S., & Strachey, J. (2001). *The complete psychological works of Sigmund Freud vol. 22: New introductory lectures on psycho-analysis & other works* (Vol. 22). Random House.

Lacan, Jacques. (1955). *Book V. The seminar of Jacques Lacan*. AFI.

Lacan, Jacques. (2011). *The seminar of Jacques Lacan: Book X: Anxiety: 1962–1963*. AFI.

Steiner, J. (2022). A theory of psychic retreats. In S. Finkelstein, and H. Weiss (Eds.), *The claustro-agoraphobic dilemma in psychoanalysis* (pp. 113–125). Routledge.

UNHCR - The UN Refugee Agency (2024). https://www.unhcr.org

Winnicott, D. W. (2016). *The collected works of DW Winnicott* (Vol. 12). Oxford University Press.

Chapter 10

The Crisis of Group Identity During the War

Experience of Working with the Ukrainian Jewish Community

Olena Slobodianiuk and Olena Osypenko

Introduction

About a decade ago, there were numerous statements regarding the fact that we were supposedly living in the most peaceful period on planet Earth (2012). However, this fact does not alleviate the pain of witnessing wars emerge during this seemingly serene period of the highest level of civilization development, where one human destroys another and their well-being in the cruelest ways imaginable. Despite the progress of humanity and its distance from primal ancestors, people still resort to savage and brutal primitive methods for annihilation.

It was during such a time, in early 2022 at the beginning of the second wave of escalation of the war in Ukraine, initiated by Russia in 2014, that all of us working as psychoanalysts heard the sounds of explosions outside our windows (Velykodna et al., 2024). We came together as a united group to explore the new experience thrust upon us. We gathered to investigate what happened to us, our analyses, and Freudian urges toward life and death. Essentially, we had nothing else left. We needed to understand what occurred and how to navigate the new realities, finally named a full-scale war. Additionally, we had to comprehend how we could now help ourselves and our analyses.

Since October 10, 2022, Russia has initiated mass shelling of critical infrastructure, resulting in the destruction of objects supplying electricity, water, and heat to homes. This period marked the emergence of a new English word, unfamiliar to us until now – "a blackout." This word can be considered a neologism for the Ukrainian language, signifying the total lack of control over one's life, approaching the limits of survival, and reverting to primitive existence. Indeed, it was so. No one could work as all jobs were electricity-dependent, and electricity was intermittently cut off for

DOI: 10.4324/9781032660257-11

4–8 hours, then restored for 2–4 hours, and the cycle repeated. The state attempted to make the outages predictable, but it proved challenging. People cooked in modern high-rise buildings by candlelight, walked up 30 floors multiple times a day, and hospitals operated on generators in emergency mode. In terms of working conditions, the absence of communication and the internet was the most challenging aspect. The well-established model of psychoanalytic online work developed over six months faced new trials. Analysts in Ukraine had to work in a constant search for an internet connection and operate from their cars (Yakushko & Meehan, 2023). It was the most difficult and unstable moment in our lives, mirrored by all the companies in Ukraine. Planning, promising, and fulfilling agreements were impossible. We could only hope that the agreements made would still materialize. Meeting reschedules became the norm, as well as cancellations due to disruptions in communication. Everyone was grateful when a meeting could take place. We operated in a mode of mental activity from the beginning of the war – "at least we have this one thing," and during the blackout, this became the fundamental logic of survival.

Launching Group Meetings

At this moment, on the 250th day of the war, a charitable organization (CO) approached me with a request to address the work process, as subordinates began sabotaging communication with the management but did not quit their jobs. The negotiation process took two months, reflecting the underlying issue for which they sought assistance.

One of the authors of this chapter, Olena Slobodianiuk, had worked with this organization for two years prior to the full-scale invasion and was familiar with their work processes. In Ukraine, several Jewish COs assist Jewish families in difficult circumstances. The CO Olena Slobodianiuk worked with specifically assists children from Jewish families in various challenging life situations – medical treatment, education, recreational activities for children with special needs, and legal aid. The organization operated smoothly and inspiringly before the war, with coordinators of charitable programs closely collaborating with religious centers. Coordinators would approach religious centers, share their work, and seek those in need of assistance. Mandatory communication with rabbis and participation in religious events were part of coordinators' work before the full-scale invasion. The CO's leader in Ukraine also supervised education, provided psychological support, and conducted supervision of workers. A significant part of their spiritual life involved periodic gatherings of all coordinators in Ukraine for communication, experience exchange, and participation in religious celebrations. As coordinators themselves put it, it was "joyful and inspiring," making them feel like members of one big family.

With the onset of the full-scale invasion, this CO underwent structural changes in its operations, similar to many other organizations in Ukraine. Each organization suffered losses for various reasons, but the crucial aspect was whether the organization could find resources for adaptation, or conversely, whether new stress exacerbated the existing crisis. Currently, it can be said that the problem that was deeply rooted in awareness was simultaneously always on the surface.

The leader described the problem as follows: before the war, she was like a "mother," and all coordinators were like "her children." They came to her with any issues they couldn't handle, both work-related and personal. The coordinators themselves worked with a large group, ranging from a few dozen to 50 people, providing assistance. Regular meetings were held between coordinators and the leader, where they reported on their work progress, sought help in challenging cases, and shared assistance and experiences. With the onset of the full-scale invasion, the flow of charitable activities for the leader to process increased exponentially. She couldn't manage processes as intimately and attentively as before. At the same time, coordinators helped evacuate some families to other countries. Some coordinators also left and abandoned their work duties. The work they used to do became impossible, and at times unnecessary. In the first month, everyone was at home feeling lost, but then the humanitarian aid flow increased, and the leader engaged in a new additional humanitarian project. Every coordinator, old and new alike, worked tirelessly day and night. However, over time, coordinators stopped communicating. The old metaphor proposed by the leader about identifying with the "loving and sacrificial Jewish queen Esther" no longer worked.

We proposed a model in which we created two workgroups of eight coordinators each, with a leading psychoanalyst and co-analyst in each group. The groups met twice a week for three weeks.

The organization itself formed the composition of the two groups, suggesting separating two opportunistic coordinators into different groups. Each group included members of the general coordinator team, who initially disagreed with "wasting" valuable time on "empty" conversations. Colleagues convinced them to attend the first meeting.

Clinical Illustration 1

The meeting in the first group began, and almost all participants were crying with happiness to see each other. These were women from different regions of Ukraine – Kyiv, Chernihiv, and Western Ukraine. They were glad to have the opportunity to see and hear their colleagues, who were truly like members of one family to them. It was very emotional and touching. Everyone complained about the terrible living conditions, and at the same time, they said that it wasn't scary, and they were overcoming everything. They were concerned for others, not just for themselves. It was as if people who had long been hiding in basements and apartments had come out into the open field and warmed each other with the rays of kindness from their hearts. At the same time, an enormous cloud is approaching from afar, carrying pain, irritation, and the thunder of discontent. In regions where there was a change in living conditions and military actions, coordinators showed support and were in an assembled state. And precisely in the regions where everything was quiet, where there were no changes in living conditions, thunder and the lightning of emotions resounded. The reason for this state turned out to be an extraordinary burden on one person due to an extremely large number of internally displaced members of the Jewish community.

One of the coordinators was consumed by anger. The number of people in her community increased tenfold. And the amount of work increased dozens and even hundreds of times, as now, not only some children needed help, but everyone who fled from explosions and war became recipients of aid. The situation changed almost overnight and lasted for ten months. She is being demanded by the rabbi and her leader to "make everyone satisfied," but she doesn't have enough blankets for all the displaced, and at the same time, she has to leave those who are close friends and with whom she has lived all her life without assistance. She knows for sure that they are not displaced persons, but they urgently need help. Internally displaced persons behave demanding and uncompromising, insisting on the assistance "they are entitled to by birthright" and should be provided. "I would be able to distribute any number of blankets, but they are not available, and they are shouting at me!"

Two circumstances became particularly difficult for this coordinator – the aggressive non-acceptance of the words "no," "there is none," and pressure and persistence of demands from both sides. The woman found herself between a rock and a hard place. On one side, the rabbi insists that everyone be satisfied, on the other side, there were demanding community members. And at this time, the person she always relied on – the NGO director – became busy with a more important task of processing humanitarian aid, for which there is no one to translate to. The country's life changed, the life of the NGO leader changed, and the lives of coordinators changed. They had to handle things on the ground. The above-mentioned circumstances were also exacerbated by personal hardship or tragedy for each person who suffered from their own misfortunes. Some had chronic illnesses exacerbated, and they needed help and treatment on their own. Someone's husband joined the military, and these people also needed support. Some had their children leave the country, leaving the person alone. Some experienced an exacerbation of the fear of losing income and employment due to the war. Some had family problems intensified because all families had to reorganize during the first days of the war and find the most acceptable new form of existence in new conditions, which sometimes meant living together in one dwelling for people of three or even four generations. All these processes were previously resolved in a religious environment and in working relationships with the leader. The function of joint reflection on situations that arose during the work process and in personal life before the war was performed willingly and extremely skillfully by the leader. With the start of the war, everything changed, and she did not realize that she had lost contact and trust with her colleagues.

Moreover, the main theme at the beginning of the first meeting was the recognition that none of the people present could control their own lives and work, could plan the future not only distant, not only tomorrow but even the next few hours. This brought everyone back to the "here and now," and there was a great longing for the past when they could plan and control. They shared they were learning to enjoy the moment, and it was a sincere truth. A cup of coffee is all that can be controlled.

Analysis of the First Group

Initially, the transfer to therapists was primarily parental. In most cases, it was positive and extremely negative among coordinators from the Western regions of Ukraine and Mykolaiv. The coordinator from Western Ukraine did not disclose all the circumstances, withheld information, and attacked requests to teach the aggressive interlocutor to say "no." She demanded demonstrations of knowledge, essentially seeking acknowledgment of helplessness and castration. She insisted on recognizing that the situation of war and extremely limited resources confronts us with the fact that we are not all-powerful, we cannot help everyone, save everyone, and ultimately, we are castrated from birth. Colleagues in more stable conditions or environments rushed to help and formed horizontal connections, offering their strengths to those in need.

The next step was reflection on the desire for omnipotence and the sense of guilt. Coordinators tried to do all the work that existed. There was a lot of work, and they exhausted themselves, experiencing poor sleep and disrupted eating behavior – some lost their appetite, while others experienced the opposite. Women started falling asleep on the go, and an extraordinary symptom was the acceleration of perception in coordinators. They did not have time to type messages and began dictating them, which they hadn't done before. They spoke faster, listened to messages at twice the speed. Certainly, this pace took its toll, and they became more nervous about children and shelling, exerting more control where it wasn't necessary. Everyone began reflecting on professional burnout, violating life sustainability norms. Braking processes did not work, but as soon as this conversation took place, they realized where they were, as their "professional mother" had taken good care of them before. They were taught how to restore their psychological state, began sharing experiences, and started caring about analytics in transfer.

In subsequent meetings, the number of attendees decreased. There were fewer expectations for learning from the analyst, and they themselves turned to their work processes and their wards. They began questioning why the mothers of their wards' children might not want to help their child when the organization offers them such an opportunity for free. They described a case where their NGO provides a service of free child treatment, but the mother does not take advantage of this opportunity. The mother behaves passively, lacking funds to treat the children and not using the provided opportunity. I think this unfolded as a fear that they were confused about their leadership, and they needed help making sense of the extraordinary experience of abandonment and vulnerability they all experienced at that moment.

The history of Jewry in Ukraine, particularly in Kyiv, has extremely painful aspects. Eighty years ago, during the German occupation of Kyiv in 1941–1943, in the Babyn Yar ravine, German occupiers executed approximately 34,000 Jews in two days – based on ethnic characteristics, as well as party and Soviet activists, underground fighters. This tragedy is part of the Holocaust – a deliberate policy of the Nazi regime to exterminate ethnic and social groups in Europe based on their racial, ethnic, national identity.

In the penultimate meetings, one of the discussion topics was whether it was advisable and safe for all coordinators to gather for a large corporate meeting where they could talk, celebrate a religious holiday, relax, receive support, and rebuild the connection that hadn't disappeared but had become like a sieve – porous and unreliable. These meetings always inspired them. In wartime, it was extremely dangerous; a "good mother" would not subject her children to even minimal risk. In understanding and modeling this situation, the group had two possible scenarios – "a good mother" thinking it's dangerous and not worth risking, and "a good father" thinking that danger always exists and careful preparation is needed.

At the last meeting, there were even fewer people. Mental stabilization was becoming evident. One of the centers was exceptionally active and had already organized a trip outside the city for a religious holiday. The coordinator was in contact with the bus in which they all traveled for the celebration. Life was overcoming death and fear.

The recent meetings clarified the expression "by birthright." The NGO provides assistance to Jewish children. But who is considered Jewish? Assistance could be given to children whose parents could confirm their Jewish affiliation for two generations through the maternal line. Before the war, not all children could enter a specialized senior school, not all could receive assistance. And since life was peaceful, it did not attract much attention. This selection did not question the survival of these children and their families. It perhaps only triggered envy and resentment for being treated as "not genuine," leading to questions about identity formation. "Who am I? Am I Jewish or Ukrainian? My father is Jewish, and my mother is Ukrainian. For Ukrainians, I am Jewish, and I am not one of them; for Jews, I am Ukrainian and half-blood." And now the individual faces the choice that exists and does not exist.

The last thought was about the fate of Jews in World War II. Acknowledging injustice from both outsiders and one's own community.

The theme of identification was raised by the coordinator from Western Ukraine, discussing that community members who evacuated from the eastern part of Ukraine, where military actions were taking place, in their identifications related to the part of the psyche that considered itself Ukrainian, did not support rituals that were dear to those who hosted them. They did not seek to celebrate common holidays; they celebrated their own, such as the holidays of the Soviet era (1917–1991), and traditions linking them to a past they no longer knew. The youth celebrated the anniversary of the pioneer organization, which was created in 1922 during Soviet times and currently does not exist in Ukraine. Their parents knew this history and were connected to their past. Celebrating Soviet holidays caused great pain to those who provided assistance. The evacuees isolated themselves with these celebrations, building a strong wall between the worlds of the west and east, demonstrating the unnecessary need for good treatment from their hosts, and at the same time, demanding acceptance and good treatment due to the "the birthright." The narcissistic trauma of the evacuees did not allow them to become friendly members of the community and set them against the local residents. The identification as "Jew" did not work, as displaced individuals faced numerous demands and aggression, and the identification as Ukrainian was replaced by Soviet identification.

According to Kernberg (1998), positive relationships among organization members depend on their mutual identification with a common task and their identification with a specific professional group. These libidinal connections also depend on transference onto their leader and enthusiasm for him (Freud, 1921). At the same time, since all human relationships are ambivalent, and organization members are especially vulnerable to rivalry due to professional advancement and administrative hierarchy, the potential for aggression also becomes important in the social life of the organization. In addition, along with idealization and dependence on their leaders, individual members demonstrate pre-Oedipal and Oedipal conflicts with parental authority. These conflicts are usually submerged and controlled by the reality of the shared task in work groups, according to Bion (Bion, 1961).

When the work ended, we requested feedback on our work, and it was extremely positive. The team of coordinators worked harmoniously. Restructuring of the NGO's work took place, and the coordinators returned to the organizational work model. The negative transference of the two coordinators did not find a solution at that time, but it decreased significantly, allowing them to function in those conditions, worry less about what they could not change, and work on new ideas.

During the work of the analytical groups, they were constantly supervised in our main working group, which allowed us to withstand pressure and attacks from angered participants and contain their affect.

The collective expectation of the coordinators from the leader as a maternal figure, that she would not abandon her maternal duty during wartime and would increase attention due to the threat of danger, did not materialize. The collective expressed its dissatisfaction with the refusal to maintain necessary communication – "You abandoned us, and we will abandon you."

The leadership called on psychotherapists to perform the parental function – establish symbolic order not through fantasy expectations of mother-child interaction, not through maternal sacrifice, but through turning to oneself and one's own resources, taking a working position where they can take care of themselves and other people. It is also important to recognize the fact that we cannot achieve everything we dream of, but we can try to do it without blaming the Other for the metaphoric castration.

Clinical Illustration 2

The second group consisted in full of women aged 30 to 70 from Kyiv, Zaporizhzhia, Mykolaiv, Odesa, Zhytomyr, Khmelnytskyi, and Tel Aviv (Israel). It was their first video meeting in nine months since the start of the full-scale war in Ukraine. All participants were tense and hesitant to start speaking.

A coordinator from Kyiv complained that since the beginning of the war, the workload has increased tens of times, the community has grown in numbers, but the team doing the work remains the same. In Ukraine, there is a blackout, but reports on the work performed need to be submitted on time. Despite the difficulties, the coordinator tries to find ways to carry out the work. All the pre-war means of working are shattered; they cannot function during the war. Now the coordinator tries to find comfort even in trivial things, for example, "I don't wear tight shoes anymore, although I used to wear such shoes before the war. Planning is a sensitive subject for me. Everything has to be scheduled and planned; I keep a diary. Now, due to the war, it doesn't work. Making plans is difficult for me now, and I try to let go and not make them. When my plans fall apart I get very upset."

A coordinator from Mykolaiv mentioned that before the war, she was involved in a project with children. Since the beginning of the war, she has been forced to handle everything: children, medical care, escorting the elderly. Mykolaiv has been under constant shelling for eight months, and the Jewish community is struggling to survive. There is no water; we have not bathed for two months, no electricity, they provide light for only an hour and a half, shellings happen at 12:00 AM, 3:00 AM, and 5:00 AM, and you sleep in between them. The main problem is that people needing help are in the corridor, and we (coordinators) need the help of psychologists to know how to help people when we ourselves are not psychologists. Therefore, she is skeptical about our meetings, wondering if it is possible to spend an hour and a half a day and how it will affect if the light and internet turn on after an hour and a half. And then she continued to share examples of horrors that happened in the community.

A bomb hit a house where a family of five lived: mother, father, grandmother, grandfather, and an 11-year-old boy. All the adults were killed; they pulled the living boy out from under the rubble, whose bladder seized to function properly due to shock; he peed himself all the time. The psychologist they turned to for help couldn't handle the mental load and cried instead of providing help. Coordinators were outraged by the psychologist's behavior. They hint at the same inability to endure their pain in the analysis of their group.

Every day lonely elderly people, abandoned by their relatives, come to the community center for food. In their eyes there is one desire – "don't abandon me." Coordinators talk about the ambivalence of their feelings – they want more than anything not to be abandoned, but they do not agree on a weak Other.

New coordinators are more peaceful and seek to collaborate with psychologists and see them as support.

One coordinator, who has been in Israel since the first days of the war, speaks of the feeling of "a stolen life, helplessness, shattered plans, and the guilt of not being present." It's difficult for her to communicate with those who stayed in Ukraine. She talks about the aggression she saw, how people get irritated, an emotional breakdown.

> I get it because at 7 AM on February 24, my only thought was - children should not see this! Save all the children you can! But I see that my children, these children of war, are very sad, living a past life, they know how life in Ukraine has changed, I talk to them, but they don't want to live abroad. After the war, children want to return home, and I had to say very harshly that we will not return to Ukraine; children must live on, develop.

The Mykolaiv coordinator immediately tried to deflect onto the psychologist, attacking the setting (the stable conditions necessary for researching and transforming mental phenomena, especially those related to the unconscious, in a special therapeutic environment), thereby hiding the impossibility of playing the role of God. The coordinator tried to change the time and day of the meeting, and after the second meeting, when the psychologist refused to meet her demand, she left the group. She attacked the analyst with direct questions: "How to distribute humanitarian aid that came in less quantity than needed?" and thus forced the analyst to take responsibility for her own helplessness.

An Israeli coordinator explained that in the Jewish community, it is customary so that no one remains unheard, without attention, support, or help. This philosophy has been ingrained in Jews for centuries. The community unconditionally provides any support. Unconditional support and love are what all members of the community expected.

In all subsequent meetings, the group discussed family relationships, anxiety due to "blackouts," chronic stress, fear of the future, the sadness and grief of not being able to turn back time. All women complained about the feeling of "suspended life."

Analysis of the Second Group

According to Foulke's (1975) theory, the natural "web" in which each occupies an individual position is the family. Additionally, each individual will resist any changes using all means available, attempting to establish a grid similar to the one they grew up in, the grid of their parental family. This inclination manifested in one participant who sought to change the group meeting time above all, disregarding the circumstances of other participants. Her argument, that it was inconvenient for her due to a conflicting event, was made despite her ability to influence that other event easily.

Another participant from the second group conveyed helplessness and fear of not handling work, echoing her inability to expect support in her own family. In her own family, she tried to assume the role of the family's head, guiding all generations out of love and fulfilling their desires. Giving up this position meant losing power and acknowledging her weakness. However, she didn't have to do this in the group, as participants who had moved abroad showed empathy and a sense of guilt for leaving Ukraine, providing their own resources to help this participant.

None of the participants from both groups dared to directly address feelings of abandonment by the leader and the increased workload. They refrained from discussing symbolic mothers and fathers who left them, appearing weak and expecting help from their children. They shifted to manic defenses like "we can distribute plenty of bread, blankets, and medicine," emphasizing that the Other cannot provide these resources for themselves and completely withdrew from contact. These defenses aimed to avoid acknowledging their own vulnerability and total castration.

The regression observed in both groups affected specific members, allowing those not in dire straits to support those who were. They proposed not blaming anyone but finding a way to solve the issues.

During group work, in crisis situations, the group regresses from a working group to a "fight-or-flight" group. The coordinator from Mykolaiv demonstrated this dynamic as she fought against injustice at work, injustice in war, and injustice in her own life. The analysts contemplated temporarily removing her from the group for individual therapy and then reintegrating her.

The analyst sought regular supervision and observed group dynamics. Group dynamics are tracked through specific elements of people's behavior within the group's dynamics. This person-marker tells us about the group's problem, just as a child reveals family problems. A mother comes to a psychoanalyst complaining about a child's bad behavior, but when the child is brought in, they turn out to be wonderful, gentle, and smart. The analyst cannot replace the child's parents but can adapt the child, teaching them to deal with difficult circumstances differently if possible.

This situation in group work is related to an identity crisis, a narcissistic issue where the individual overvalues their importance, seeks constant recognition, and considers themselves superior to others. The existential threat is triggered by aggression and external conditions, causing a sense of danger and a narcissistic crisis. According to Freud (1921), libido returns to the ego, and the person is temporarily unable to invest in objects. Frustrated drives also awaken internal aggression, manifested in attacks on the analyst. In better times, this aggression is contained, channeled into acceptable aggression, or sublimated into creative activities. However, external aggression and life-threatening situations induce fear, absorb mental energy, and test our weakest defense mechanisms.

Of course, in such moments, it is more challenging to overcome and transform the patient's aggression. The analyst may be all-powerful in the patient's fantasies, which usually cannot be compared to reality. In these groups, a fantasy was expressed that "the mother" sent analysts to watch over "the children" and report on their behavior, which participants believed.

Participants shifted to a fantasy of an all-powerful father with support from religion. They began planning religious celebrations. Others recognized the need to care for their charges to feel stronger themselves, nurturing the identity of "the benefactor." They understood that this identity was dictated not only by the needs of the current situation but also by a much deeper necessity.

Conclusion

The danger, helplessness, shock, and chaos discussed by the group leader as a significant third member of the therapeutic dyad group-analyst can be considered. As long as it remains externalized, a separate "object" beyond the interaction of the dyad, we cannot do anything with it. It should be introduced into the dyad and treated as a third element. The dyad does not create a rigid connection against the external enemy – reality. It must allow this "essence" into its territory and give it a worthy place in the therapeutic setting, as rejected reality returns in aggression against those who try not to notice it.

The dynamic interaction of libidinal and aggressive impulses occurs not only in the dynamic unconscious of the individual but also at the group level. Defensive and sublimation processes expressing the vicissitudes of libido and aggression can be observed at both individual and group levels, and their activation depends on circumstances and the individual characteristics of the group leader, his ability to recognize reality and his own mental strengths.

According to McWilliams (2021), the supervisor plays a crucial role in helping the analyst endure the suffering of his patients when it comes to an experience that cannot be changed. Working with groups occurred in such challenging conditions and required so much mental effort that relying on the supervisor alone made it possible. Although sadness never completely fades (Pavlovska, 2023), over time it becomes easier for a person, and the process of experiencing grief enriches those who have been able to go through it.

References

Bion, W. R. (1961). *Experiences in groups and other papers*, Tavistock, London.

Foulkes, S. H. (1975). *Group-analytic psychotherapy. Method and principles*. Gordon and Breach.

Freud, S. (1921). *Massenpsychologie und Ich-Analyse*. Internationaler Psychoanalytischer Verlag.

Kernberg, O. F. (1998). *Ideology, conflict, and leadership in groups and organizations*. Yale University Press.

McWilliams, N. (2021). *Psychoanalytic supervision*. Guilford Publications.

Pavlovska, O. (2023). Psychoanalytic work with losses during the war: The Ukrainian experience. *Psychoanalytic Psychology*, 40(4), 251.

Velykodna, M., Butsykin, Y., Dorozhkin, V., Lupis, A., Melnychuk, T., Nalyvaiko, N., … & Yakushko, O. (2024). Inscribing a new page in the history of Ukrainian psychoanalysis during the wartime: The call for contributions. *International Journal of Applied Psychoanalytic Studies*, 21(2), e1861.

Yakushko, O., & Meehan, K. B. (2023). Psychoanalysis and war: On witnessing Ukrainian psychoanalysts. *Psychoanalytic Psychology*, 40(4), 235.

Chapter 11

The "Severed Roots" People

Psychoanalytic Reflections from Running the Psychological Hotline Work with Ukrainian Refugees

Sergii Ugrium

Transformation and Challenges of Psychological Assistance in Wartime

The experience and reflections I share were born from the meta-event we Ukrainians call the Great War, which has unleashed a torrent of changes in the physical and emotional life of every Ukrainian. Certainly, wars are complex situations with specific effects on the inner world of every individual. In Ukraine, the war situation encouraged mental health professionals to propose initiatives to quickly and effectively address the "mental fire" that has engulfed Ukrainians. Concepts such as deep, complex, non-linear, multilayered, and long-term psychological work—the epithets familiar to our profession, especially in psychoanalytic practice—have given way to urgent psychological aid. This new reality prompted many Ukrainian psychoanalysts to make unprecedented changes in the psychotherapy process, both with their new patients as well as patients who have been engaged within what is viewed as a "standard" therapeutic setting (Dorozhkin, 2023; Lagutin, 2023; Nalyvaiko, 2023; Velykodna, 2023). Notably, no psychoanalyst in these times can ignore the relevance of acute ongoing war trauma or reduce patient issues exclusively to familiar internal conflicts and the traumatic events of childhood. In each of our patients, we now can see the images of war and its impact on the individuals' psychic foundations.

One initiative to address mental health needs during this wartime is the psychological hotline for emergency or crisis assistance, established by the National Psychological Association of Ukraine (Palii et al., 2023). The hotline combines the efforts of professionals from various psychological fields and orientations, making it possible to share experiences, observations, and findings together with colleagues across numerous theoretical traditions. The current format of the hotline is based on a one-time remote session of

DOI: 10.4324/9781032660257-12

up to one hour. Certainly, such a format is unusual and creates challenges for psychoanalytically based clinicians like myself, who are used to having a protected private space as well as sufficient time with the patients to work through their traumatic material. At times, I felt like a surgeon who was used to a meticulous, dedicated workspace for surgeries, being suddenly placed in an intensive care unit and even more challenging in a make-shift mobile medical unit. I wondered whether I could be useful in a one-time counseling format and what I could do to facilitate the creation of a supportive, safe, therapeutic container, all while I faced so much destruction and threats to life. Therefore, my reflections on this work are based on an in-depth understanding within psychoanalysis of the processes, often evident in a psychic content, that speaks to human beings on the verge of death/survival. I could also draw on my ability to hear beneath or what is not conveyed directly in words via the rational part of the discourse. I could focus on my ability to create a distinct containing space that could be relied on by patients to reduce their excessive pain and anxiety. Finally, I could engage in this work through my willingness to accept the vulnerability of our human nature and the finite nature of our being, which emphasizes the profound value of human life.

Certainly, each individual story is unique, holding distinct sets of circumstances and an unfolding life path. However, being in the midst of a war is a possibility about which most human beings rarely think about or plan for, and for which individuals are not mentally prepared. The war experience offers no standard theoretical developmental categories, identifiable algorithms, or guidelines; most humans have no rules for coping or engaging with wars. Today every Ukrainian confronts this apocalyptic situation of uncertainty and threat to life. Many Ukrainians, even if (temporarily) physically safe from Russian aggression, have relatives who had to remain in the war zones. A tremendous number of Ukrainians lost their homes, lands, or properties. Many Ukrainians endured the horrific experience of escaping to safety under active military fire. Many had to abandon everything, leaving their homes and lives in order to find somewhere safe to stay alive. Among the most striking observations I made, which I further discuss below, is how much these details and difficulties, which vary greatly, appear to be secondary to something deep and profound, which is present in almost every Ukrainian story and which often does not appear to correlate at all with how successfully a person seemed to overcome the war circumstances. As I suggest, the scale of this apocalyptic event cannot be comprehended through rational arguments or common sense, which is typically used to assess human situations. I focus on this observation throughout the chapter.

The Crisis of Life Investments in the Face of a War Migration

> I don't know how to describe my condition. I don't know what exactly worries me. I guess I am confused by my existence here. I feel like a tree that fell into a river and was carried away. It's almost impossible to understand where my legs are and where my head is. And then it's like this tree washed up on some bank, at least temporarily. I'm not even a tumbleweed, which has this nomadic nature, but just a tree with severed roots, or better yet, a half-living piece of wood that used to be a tree.

This self-reflection was shared during one of my consultations, poetically describing one of the central issues of the experiences faced by people who were forced to flee their homes in order to escape away from the frontlines, internally in Ukraine or abroad. My attention in hearing this statement was drawn not only to the contents of the experience but also to the form itself: I felt as if something large, heavy, and without a clear structure filled the inner and intersubjective space. Words we can access seem simply powerless in holding and describing what is being experienced.

Individuals who manage to verbalize their states beyond simple statements such as "I feel bad" or "Life has lost its sense" and build some connections to their mental states typically describe their primary concerns as the inability to fully adapt to new life conditions, to accept other "rules of the game," to "live in the present," to formulate plans and make connections, or to allow themselves to experience positive emotions. For them, life was put on hold without instructions or explanations. A closer study of such cases revealed to me that total maladjustment, rejection, and even attacks on the new situation are often related to manifestations and consequences of the crisis of life investments because the environment, the reality of the present, plans for the future, and the person's life itself ceased to be the primary objects of normal libidinal investments.

I view the concept of life investments as libidinal investments arising from psychic processes that serve life goals, especially the formation of object connections and social integration. This psychic life investment stands in opposition to destructive changes that play on the side of death. These concepts are connected to classic and contemporary ideas related to Eros/ Life Drive versus Thanatos/Death Drive (Gaitanidis, 2024). In general, these concepts focus on the channeling of libidinal energy, in particular the interests, attention, and aspirations, toward what fills a person's life—their location, environment, activity, plans, connections with other people, and so forth. These are also investments of the Self as an agent of solving problems and achieving desired goals. Thus, the focus is on whether a person's life is filled with actual vitality or whether it is just a mechanical existence using a kind of perverse mechanism that prevents the emergence and development of something more alive and resilient. If this vitality somehow "evaporates" from life, it is important to understand what factors contribute to its diminishment or absence.

In the context of interest in life, the very act of making self-assertion or requesting assistance is a very important step. Thus, those of us working the hotline usually emphasize this important form of life investment in a crisis conversation with a patient. The person has invested also in speaking with the other (i.e., one of us as crisis responders) who can help them locate new knowledge/information and a place within themselves for this emerging understanding. Certainly, not every person who calls the hotline expects help. In addition to the constructive options that prompt many to call in for assistance, their subconscious motivations may be different and, at times, even destructive. They can call to gain the elementary release of their problematic impulses or they call in order to re-affirm the stalemate in their situation—their hopelessness, their sense of futility in making any effort. Thus, one of the most traumatic effects of war is the breaking of links, including untying the drives of life and death, leading to the inability of Eros to restrain Thanatos, which often leads to the uncontrolled dominance of the death drive and the blocking of purposeful activities. However, in cases where there is some hope present, which is essential to life investment, supporting it is one of our main tasks in brief hotline crisis interventions.

The typical experience shared by Ukrainians displaced by war is something along the lines of "Most of all, I want to go back, but I can't right now because I have small children/a mother who needs treatment/it's not safe at all." It evokes solidarity and full understanding both on the part of the voiced (internal) desire and the (external) arguments provided. But the illusion of the imaginary is relaxed in this case, noting the shared base desire Ukrainians share, we can still engage them with questions such as "Where does the person actually want to return to?; Why does it not work out?; And how does all this affect their current mental state and adaptation?" It is in these further questions that the life investments can be examined, including what might have destroyed them and where they emerge to the surface of awareness. Notably, for many individuals, these investments are anchored to something that is no longer available. Therefore, we must recognize and work with the logic of libidinal deadlock in their experience of loss.

The Losses of War and the Peculiarities of Grief among the Classics of Psychoanalysis

The war took many things away from us. We have lost our protected space, control over our own lives, faith in tomorrow, in ourselves, our strength, and in the carefree and stable world, and much more. The social circle has changed significantly, with bitter disappointments and great discoveries. The order in which we previously existed has been overturned; the social Other no longer guarantees safety and does not give clear instructions, and we have no one to lean on when making a decision or choice. A certain pulverization of the Other as an authority is experienced, and we seek to re-discover this Other in politicians, experts, psychics, and even casual acquaintances who seem to know the "truth," psychologists among these.

The war took away our old life, what we were so used to, and what we had become attached to. This is perhaps one of the greatest tragedies and losses we will ever experience. It seems easy to say, "Forget it, let it go, the past is the past," but the work of mourning is a complex process. However, it is clear that without mourning the loss of our previous life, we will not be able to effectively invest in the present and in the future. The metapsychological understanding of this process certainly stems from Freud's (1917) well-known theory, proposed in *Mourning and Melancholia*. Freud suggested that the work of mourning carried out under the influence of the reality principle, should provide a de-cathexis of psychic energy via a gradual abandonment of the investment into an object of attachment in order to further reinvest this energy into new realities and relations. In the case of Ukrainians, viewed from our psychological observations, the desired return is often expressed as a wish to return to old life and to the situation before the war.

The pioneers of psychoanalytic theories after Freud actively employed his theories on mourning, revealing additional aspects related to the development of the grieving process. For example, Karl Abraham (2018), in his correspondence with Freud, drew attention to the manic mechanisms that may accompany loss and emphasized the increase in libido on the occasion of the loss of an object. Notably, as Ukrainian psychoanalysts, we too have observed reports of increased sexual desire in the clinic or in everyday life after a loss, which seems, at the very least, important for pain relief. This increase in the libido, observed by other psychoanalysts, can surprise the grieving person and may be experienced as a form of irreparable sin—the sin of being overwhelmed by desire, of being surprised by a libido that emerges at the most inopportune moment, when the person should be grieving (Torok, 2014). Moreover, Melanie Klein (1994) examined grief through the prism of the relationship with an early good object, the loss of which is actualized in cases of bereavement.

The Hungarian psychoanalyst Maria Torok (2014) also supported the idea that normal mania was prevalent in the experience of mourning, characterized by a short-term increase in libido. She further introduced the distinction between the processes of introjection and incorporation in this libidinal increase. Introjection, she stressed, marked the normal process of grieving and separation from the lost object by redirecting the libido away from this object into the Self in order that the libido can be redirected to newly available objects. If the desires related to the lost object were then well introjected and appropriated by the Self, then no emotional catastrophe or melancholic failure is experienced as destructive to the self and life. If the introjection is insufficient, then the installation of the forbidden (lost) object in the inner psychic space occurs, which Torok called the incorporation. In contrast to the progressive process of introjection, incorporation is aligned with more magical defensive processes and operates through hallucinatory ideations (Torok, 2014). The person whose mourning is marked by the incorporation will unconsciously seek out the "corpse" of this lost object in the hope of its subsequent resurrection.

John Steiner (2022) offers an alternative understanding of the work of mourning, in which the reality of what belongs to the object, on the one hand, and to the Self, on the other hand, is revised. As a result of this revision, the projected parts of the Self-return to their place, and the object appears in a more realistic form. This process actually repeats the model of initial object separation, which brings the grieving process closer to reaching a depressive position. In the course of mourning, a symbolic function is formed, which, in principle, allows the person to distinguish between what belongs to the Self and the other. If the subject is unable to withstand the psychic pain of loss, they resort to the formation of specific internal defensive functions called psychic retreats—protective psychic constructions built from projective identification, idealization, distortion of reality, and humble submission in order to achieve the goal of hiding from pain and suffering.

Another significant concept related to theorizing primary grief was proposed by Racamier (2016), which was based on the Object Relation theory. Racamier suggested that the Self must perform the work of mourning in relation to the narcissistic unity and refuse an absolute possession of the primary object. In fact, Racamier emphasized that the process of discovering the object, as such, may not be fully discovered or experienced before it is lost. Without mourning the object, which a person has to endure, there can be no autonomy and flourishing of the subject. Racamier notes that the intersection of primal grief allows individuals to believe in themselves and in objects and to invest in them as well as develop an ability to develop sufficient trust in the world and in life, both in the object and in oneself. In the reasoning of the above-mentioned psychoanalytic theorists, the emphasis is made (more or less) on identifiable objects, specifically the significant figures in the emotional life of a person. During the experience of a loss, or to be more precise, in the case of Ukrainian refugees and displaced individuals, multiple and profound losses that have radically changed their lives, the function of identifying loss, of singling out the objects of loss, is severely disrupted due to multiple, non-specific, dispersed, and abstract nature of loss.

Ukrainians often can name a kind of "vague objects" that are, in fact, rather formless in their substances, which they can potentially turn into objects of loss under favorable psychic conditions. The following fragment of a patient's description of their experiences is a revealing illustration of this process.

> Almost every day, in the flow of whatever tasks, I wait in vain for someone or something to return, to give me moments of joy and hope, to throw a hug around my shoulders, and inspire me to move forward. But no matter how hard I try to listen or pay attention, I can't tell what kind of a ghost it is that I'm waiting for. Maybe I'm waiting for something that doesn't exist yet, or maybe it exists in a different form to return. It's all very strange and incomprehensible.

This statement points not to a diffused feeling but to something that already has the markings of an object and can occupy a certain spatial position; it can interact with a subject for whom there is a certain longing and expectation toward it. The presence and action of this object-making function can be identified as if preparing the form for the emergence of the object—the future object of loss. In other words, in order to mourn the loss of an object, one must not only have access to it but sometimes even create it. In addition, even if it is in some sense synthetic (i.e., not original or indigenous) and appears post factum (i.e., constructed rather than reconstructed), the psyche may be able to engage with it.

The French psychoanalyst André Green (1999) developed a theory with a focus on the importance of the objectifying function, especially evident in *The Work of the Negative*. This function, Green emphasized, consists not only in the formation of relations with an object (i.e., external or internal) but also in the possibility of transforming a structure into an object. Objectification is not limited to the transformation of an object; it can elevate to the rank of an object something that has neither the qualities nor the attributes of an object (Green, 1999). Specifically, Green stressed that the movement, the transformation of "something" to the status and characteristics of an object, is possible due to the function of objectification.

Another example of such transformation occurs when an unoriginal, secondary object of loss is utilized to carry out the overall work of mourning. This process is illustrated in statements such as "there can't be happiness, but maybe misfortune helped." In one of my clinical cases, a person who was in a state of despair or faced an unformed mass of multiple losses may be able to overcome their situation by experiencing the loss of a specific love object that appeared in his life almost immediately after his traumatic relocation or escape. While at first the sadness and confusion over both finding and losing this new temporary love object were diffuse in light of numerous other losses (i.e., his psyche clearly lacked more or less defined objects to connect with), after the romantic disappointment, the pain and sadness became clearer, and the psyche could better cope with overall losses.

Rethinking the Fate of the Lost in Contemporary Psychoanalytic Thought

It seems that the work of mourning is a far more complex and nuanced process than simply redirecting investments from what was lost to what is new. Contemporary theories emphasize the formation of connections, transformation, and symbolization of the experience. In their theorizing, the object of loss does not completely disappear, does not drown in the river of oblivion, but remains present albeit transformed. This is not the resurrection of a "corpse" as suggested by Torok (2014), but giving the object a new life. Thus, in my own theorizing based on these readings and my clinical work, the work of grief is a kind of differentiation of what needs to be let go and what needs to be kept and transformed. In practical terms, I distinguish between forgetting and preserving on the one hand and transformation and symbolization on the other hand. Therefore, in the normal course of grieving, individuals can form a memory of the lost object, a sense of nostalgia, and its influence on our emotions, thoughts, and actions.

Hagman (1995) suggested that the transformation and internal restructuring of attachment to the object of loss, influenced by the experience of communication with the environment, holds potential for empathy as well as more articulated social prescriptions and restrictions. Gaines (1997) also emphasized the work of "creating continuity" in loss—the realization of two tasks of grieving, both distancing from the object of loss and forming a continuous connection with it. Kernberg (2010) proposed that as a result of grief, a permanent connection between the subject and the lost object is formed, leading to certain structural changes in the Ego and the Super-Ego. In addition to the function of blame, the latter can develop ideals and value systems that are important for personal development. Kernberg points out that the investment in new objects can be even greater, leading to an increase in love. In this case, when facing multiple losses, the experience gained will have to resonate with the requirements of the new environment. Thus, the lost object must be present within the individual but in a form that does not drain the libidinal energy, instead enriching psychic structures and stimulating the processes of integration, transformation, and symbolization.

The multiple losses that Ukrainians have endured against the backdrop of war and displacement are, of course, more complex and diffused in contrast to those losses, which are typically theorized about in psychoanalysis. By their nature, Ukrainians' losses as the result of war may be similar to intangible secondary losses that also accompany the loss of a significant person. For example, Volkan and Zintl (2018) provided examples of varied secondary losses that can be connected to a person's social position, prestige, roles, life habits, and so forth, which most Ukrainians have faced to a small or larger degree.

Role and Functions of the Other in Grief Counseling

When examining data from the hotline counseling sessions, I observed that the focus on the loss of a prior life may not appear on the surface or even be explicitly named by the crisis session clients. The loss of an entire past life appears often hidden within feelings of loss of purpose, the forfeiture of mental strength, difficulties in adaptation, an increase in negative affective states, increased generalized anxiety, or even in the attacks on one's own lifestyle and environment. However, with some clients, my colleagues and I have begun to identify the specific symptoms of grief, even within a single crisis session, and have come to the conclusion the reconfigurations of attitude toward a life to which the person can never physically return is vital. Certainly, the format of a single meeting usually allows one to adjust the optics of such perceptions, encouraging the individual toward a direction for their reflection and creation of conditions that facilitate the work of mourning. However, our experience suggests that it is not so much rational decisions, analysis of the situation, and development of adaptation skills that make the most impact in these brief single sessions. We found that the positive experience of containment is marked by warm human contact with another person who is not afraid to face someone else's pain, confusion, states of internal destruction, enormity of shame, and despair; that aids the individual in this session toward symbolization. Our capacity to contain and mirror, with warmth and care, appears to give hope to individuals we meet with only for a brief single session—hope that such supportive experiences can be repeated to others. We are neither gods nor wizards—we cannot stop the war, repair all the destruction, or eliminate suffering. Yet the unique experience of an empathetic interaction and human sensitivity, of respect and even love in some sense, an experience that has clear time limits and thus becomes very rich in what it offers, appears in many cases to breathe life into a good object space within a person, inviting them toward the stage of a radically new life.

Loss is, to a large extent, a social feeling. A number of researchers, such as Hagman (1996) and Bowlby (2008), emphasize the role of the other in the grieving process and highlight that human support is a crucially important factor in successfully going through and bearing loss. Among the functions of the other, in addition to helping to understand the reality of loss and overcome the shock, Hagman (1996) identified the importance of the containment space, in which the environment takes care of the person's needs (especially in their regressive states), satisfying libidinal needs and making libidinal objects available, providing narcissistic resources, while also modeling, containerizing, and symbolizing affect (Hagman, 1996). We found that most of these functions, especially assistance in consciously facing the loss, stimulating the expression of emotions, containing them, and translating them into words, can be realized during crisis assistance.

Difficulties and Successes of Integration and Symbolization Processes in Overcoming Loss

Displaced persons, especially those who have found themselves abroad within a radically different environment, way and pace of life, may show signs of defensive disidentification. In a sense, they cannot integrate their self-states that are based on their past and their present. I have especially observed such defensive moves as, "canceling" or devaluing their skills, experience, and knowledge. Time appears to them as warped: the fixed boundaries of memory are blurred and faded, the past only shows up in a striking and strange way, and the future has no definite image or outline. Their Self seems to be less tied to certain internal images, ideas, and feeling states (Freud, 1989); they seem to start "drifting" (Ivanova, 2023, p. 57). At the same time, their Self finds itself under extreme pressure, which can be profoundly exhausting. On the one hand, their deep narcissistic wounds are evident: being a war victim, a refugee, a person who has lost almost everything, including stable narcissistic support systems. The castrating effect of "starting from scratch" can be shocking, and there is a kind of mental splitting of life into "before" and "after" with difficulty in using the experience that is already gained. Thus, the task of the counselor often lies in bringing the person out of this state of shock and helping them identify how their existing knowledge and skills can be applied in the current situation. On the other hand, the Self appears as if captured by a haunting sense of guilt that blocks any attempts to invest in a new life and tap into an important mental resource in the form of pleasure. Personal goals fall under strict prohibitions, and only the over- and transpersonal acts begin to matter (Dorozhkin, 2023, p. 34). These splits are also expressed in the irrational fears of adaptation based on the fear "What if I like it?" This fear can nearly automatically level out previous cathexes and a person's will to choose between "here" and "there," "now" and "then." However, investing one's life in the present also implies investing it in the past, because human beings base their experiences and knowledge from sources in their past. In addition, investing in the present is a requirement for the libidinal investment also in the future because such inner work creates a kind of base for future recovery.

Clinical Case Examples and Observations

The following four brief examples, taken from consultations on the crisis hotline, are used to demonstrate different approaches to the losses, often identified by the person on an unconscious level of communication. Among these examples, I hope to illustrate both the examples of psychic stagnation as well as more successful adaptation scenarios.

The first case example, which was particularly characteristic of the beginning of mass migration by Ukiranians fleeing the horrors of war, describes a woman who crossed the borders. In the crisis session, she describes taking her belongings out of her suitcase at the beginning of each day and packing them back before going to bed. Thus, she shows (rather than tells) her expectation of not staying in the new location for a long time. Her unpacking and packing is a metaphor for the preservation of her past experience and knowledge while also pointing to the avoidance of the integration into her current situation. This pattern also resonates with the use of psychic retreats in the formulations by Steiner (2022), mentioned earlier. The person with the suitcase denies the fact of her existence in a changed reality, where it is necessary to unpack her belongings (her libidinal investments) and to find new places for them.

This second example demonstrates a transformational process. A Ukrainian refugee woman described how every Sunday, she and her children actively sought out experiences in nature in their new country. She noted that this tradition carried over from her life in Ukraine in their hometown. Thus, a person can actualize their habitual pattern of behavior, in different conditions. Moreover, this client described her experiences through the prism of enriching (adding to) herself and her children with new impressions of another place.

The third example illustrates the formation of symbols that may be important in the work of mourning. A woman I met with stated that when she was little, her grandmother often wore a beautiful blue embroidered (Ukrainian) dress during the holidays, which was a cherished memory because it was associated with moments of joy and happiness. While abroad, the woman suddenly decided that she should have a similar blue dress. She then described her profound surprise when she saw almost the exact same dress in a foreign store and bought it. Certainly, the point of this case is not that she bought a similar dress in the literal sense but that, first of all, she invested, within her mental space, in the process of mourning, which may have aided her in holding on to a good object and a positive past experience.

Finally, I wish to share an example that I particularly liked and which I experienced as an example of a psychological discovery. The case involved writing letters to the self in the past. In these letters, the person described their present life, experiences, and difficulties, referring to images in the past as the Other. In one such example, a woman shared a letter in which she wrote, "Remember, your husband taught you to ride a bicycle, so today I finally understood what all those scratched knees were for."

In conclusion, undoubtedly each human beings, especially when facing the war, find their individual unique way to integrate their experience, to symbolize their losses, and to understand that despite great changes and significant challenges, they can retain the core of their personality. Even in horror war conditions, human beings can hold on to the core of their being, which indeed strives to live no matter what.

References

Abraham, K. (2018). *The complete correspondence of Sigmund Freud and Karl Abraham 1907–1925*. Routledge.

Bowlby, E. J. M. (2008). *Loss-sadness and depression: Attachment and loss volume 3*. Random House.

Dorozhkin, V. (2023). Current war and its impact on the therapeutic relationship. *Ukrainian Psychoanalytic Journal*, 1(1), 32–35. https://doi.org/10.32782/upj/2023-1-6

Freud, S. (1917). Mourning and melancholia. *The Standard Edition of the Complete Psychological Works of Sigmund Freud*, 14(1914–1916), 237–258.

Freud, S. (1989). *Inhibitions, symptoms, and anxiety*. WW Norton & Company.

Gaines, R. (1997). Detachment and continuity: The two tasks of mourning. *Contemporary Psychoanalysis*, 33(4), 549–571.

Gaitanidis, A. (2024). The death drive revisited: a relational psychoanalytic perspective. *Ukrainian Psychoanalytic Journal*, 2(3), 43–50. https://doi.org/10.32782/upj/2024-2-3-5

Green, A. (1999). *The work of the negative*. Free Association Books.

Hagman, G. (1995). Mourning: A review and reconsideration. *The International Journal of Psycho-Analysis*, 76(5), 909.

Hagman, G. (1996). The role of the other in mourning. *The Psychoanalytic Quarterly*, 65(2), 327–352.

Ivanova, L. (2023). Dynamics of mental processes during periods of crises, grief, and rites of passage based on calculations of psychological defense mechanisms. *Ukrainian Psychoanalytic Journal*, 1(3), 56–65. https://doi.org/10.32782/upj/2023-3-9

Kernberg, O. (2010). Some observations on the process of mourning. *The International Journal of Psychoanalysis*, 91(3), 601–619.

Klein, M. (1994). 9. Mourning and its relation to manic-depressive States. *Essential Papers on Object Loss*, 1, 95.

Lagutin, V. (2023). Psychoanalysis "Traumatized" by war. Four clinical illustrations of the vulnerability of the setting. *Ukrainian Psychoanalytic Journal*, 1(3), 18–23. https://doi.org/10.32782/upj/2023-3-3

Nalyvaiko, N. (2023). Language metamorphoses as representations of subjectivity. Ukraine. Dairy of war. *Ukrainian Psychoanalytic Journal*, 1(1), 27–31. https://doi.org/10.32782/upj/2023-1-5

Palii, V., Velykodna, M., Pereira, M., Mcelvaney, R., Bernard, S., Klymchuk, V., … Gómez-Maquet, Y. (2023). The experience of launching a psychological hotline across 21 countries to support ukrainians in wartime. *Mental Health and Social Inclusion*. https://doi.org/10.1108/MHSI-04-2023-0040

Racamier, P. C. (2016). *Le Deuil Originaire*. Paris: Payot.

Steiner, J. (2022). A theory of psychic retreats. In S. Finkelstein, and H. Weiss (Eds.), *The claustro-agoraphobic dilemma in psychoanalysis* (pp. 113–125). Routledge.

Torok, M. (2014). The Illness of mourning and the 19 fantasy of the exquisite corpse. In A. Margulies (Ed.), *Reading French psychoanalysis* (pp. 388–404). Routledge.

Velykodna, M. (2023). Russia's war against Ukraine and some issues of psychoanalytic training. *Ukrainian Psychoanalytic Journal*, 1(1), 47–53. https://doi.org/10.32782/upj/2023-1-8

Volkan, V. D., & Zintl, E. (2018). *Life after loss: The lessons of grief*. Routledge.

Chapter 12

Psychoanalytic Therapy with Children in the Realities of War

An Analysis That Cannot Be

Yelyzaveta Davoian, Daria Kyrylova, and Zoia Miroshnyk

We wish to begin this chapter on working with children with a childhood-related analogy that is familiar to all of us. When children learn to ride a bicycle, they start with extra training wheels to learn to keep balance and keep from falling. Learning to ride or riding becomes impossible if either the training wheels or the regular wheels break. The Russian war in Ukraine is not only destroying human lives, including the lives of many children, but is also damaging the foundation of children's lives. Most of us as child psychoanalysts in Ukraine have been or remain under continual mortal danger, which for many of our child and family patients is yet another attack on the structures that uphold their lives. In addition, as we discuss below, in conditions of war many parents experience a significant reductions in their capacity to support their children (both physically and psychically), often projecting into or demanding from children certain responses, especially via mechanisms of guilt, which we believe can further undermine child's "wheels" of balance. In this contribution we discuss how these conditions further create an attack on psychoanalytic being-with and space in working with children and families. Moreover, we as Ukrainian child psychoanalysts also view this reality as a call to further response and shift in working with parents who may (often unconsciously and in defense-driven ways) limit the capacity for their children to develop psychic subjectivity.

Impossibility of Meeting in Psychoanalysis with Children in War-Time Ukraine

In an introduction to our chapter, we begin with a brief background. In 2019, Ukraine, like the whole world, was seized by the COVID-19 pandemic. It was in the midst of this crisis that we understood that psychoanalytic work

DOI: 10.4324/9781032660257-13

can also be conducted remotely. Adult analysands, albeit with difficulties, accepted the reality that further work, based on safety considerations, should take place remotely, but the questions remained regarding working with young analysands. After all, in psychoanalysis with children, we use various additional therapeutic means—drawing, sculpting, playing—which are difficult to implement through the computer or telephone screen. Fortunately, with time, we learned to use protective equipment, disinfectants, masks, and vaccinations, which allowed us to meet children safely in the office. Work continued. Little by little, everyone adapted to the conditions of the pandemic, and we began to move toward removing the limitations imposed on our lives by COVID-19. Ukraine and the world were gradually recovering from the pandemic and returning to their usual course of things.

Before the full-scale military invasion of Ukraine by the Russian Federation, there were many different kinds of media reports about the possible start of hostilities: news sources provided reports, bloggers commented, but, in general, varied global and local authorities denied the scenario that would include a full-scale military attack. Therefore, for several weeks or months, Ukrainians lived in a state of strong fear as well as in denial of the reality of their fear. During this period, we noticed a change in the nature of requests to us as psychoanalytic child specialists. The number of requests from parents of teenagers and teenagers themselves regarding the management of low mood states, anxiety, phobias, and depressive symptoms increased. When we met in the office with our young patients, we discovered that changes in these symptoms corresponded with psychotic states that were present in society at large.

However, we observed that both our teen patients and we, as analysts, benefited from meeting directly in the offices (unlike in COVID), which brought an intersubjective sense of security and stability. Yet this state did not last long: on February 24, 2022, at 4 o'clock in the morning, Russia launched a full-scale invasion of Ukraine, and we all woke up with sounds of air raids and explosions that covered various cities of our country.

Life stopped. The first thing we did was to ask our relatives and analysands if everything was OK with them and if they were safe. The next step was the question of whether to go to work. Will we be able to ensure safety in our office for the analysands because masks, sanitizers, and vaccination cannot save us from a missile strike? Therefore, it was decided to postpone the scheduled sessions for a week. Initially, we were hoping that the attack was some kind of misunderstanding that would be resolved in a week. But after a week, the work had to be postponed for another week and then another. In many cases, either the connection with the analysands was lost, or the work was stopped due entirely to the impossibility of conducting sessions safely.

Military events, without a doubt, profoundly influenced both our patients as and us as analysts. In order to save their lives, many people fled abroad, including many psychoanalysts. In addition to adapting to these war conditions, we also had to adapt to the living circumstances of being in a front-line city where the Russian troops and attacks were active. Certainly, this reality delayed the return to work with our patients. The opportunity to resume practice appeared only after a certain period of time when some sense of safety could be assured. However, then we encountered new and unexpected obstacles in psychoanalytic practice, which prompted our reflections on psychoanalysis with children in wartime conditions. Our experience of working in these changed conditions created an impression that our analysis was no longer possible.

Calls began from parents who sought out psychological work for their children and became very frequent. Yet after the initial connection and request, the work often never started, because it seemed that it was enough for many parents to simply let someone hear about their request (we discuss this pattern below). Often, having waited to meet our patients for the first time in the office, they would not show up. Typically, they neither came nor made any further contact. In addition, at times, they would make it to the initial session only never to return, as if a single contact was sufficient for them at that moment in their lives. Certainly, psychoanalytic work was not possible for many to engage with.

In this chapter, we will try to share the experience of psychoanalytic work with children during the war in a front-line city. We raise the question of why and what type of psychoanalysis cannot take place in such circumstances. We present our experiences via a case by one of the authors (Davoian), whose two-session treatment is illustrative of how and why psychoanalytic practice with children under conditions of war faces numerous impossibilities.

Clinical Illustration

In preparing this case for publication, we decided to give it a title of "I'm Afraid of (Your) Aggression." The case focuses on two sessions with a child who was brought into treatment at the beginning of 2023 (almost a year following the invasion) by a mother who sought help for what she described as instances of aggression by her 10-year-old son (here named R). She and her child recently returned to Ukraine from another European country, where they spent almost a year as refugees. When asked to join in the first session together with the child's father, it was made clear that both the child's biological and stepfather were not available to join but supported his treatment. In addition, R's mother shared that the stepfather, to whom R was close, was now involved in the military defense of Ukraine, which caused R considerable fears and worries. Mother specifically expressed concerns about how her son's symptoms were related to R's extreme worries for his step-father.

In our initial session, when R came in with his mother, he appeared excited and curious about the analytic office and the toys present there. During the initial meeting, when R was asked directly about why he thought he was in the psychologist's office, he replied he knew that he acted out and that his mother did not like his behavior. He seemed to know he was brought in for psychological help but did not know what it entailed.

Notably, confusion about mental health professionals is common for most Ukrainians. During the seven-decade Soviet occupation, many Ukrainians combined and confused outpatient psychology with inpatient psychiatry, often knowing that these occupations were involved not only in "mental health" but also in control and abuse of individuals whose ideas deviated from rigid Soviet norms. In addition, psychoanalysis was officially forbidden. However, since the liberation of Ukraine and its declaration of independence in 1991, psychology and psychoanalysis have become more familiar and understandable to the general public following years of education and public information campaigns. Still, like most psychoanalysts worldwide, we also have to introduce to our patients the specifics of analytic work as well as the therapeutic frame, including confidentiality.

In this session, R expressed feelings that while he was not sure what psychological help was about, he was uneasy to be left alone without his mother in the office because he did not seem informed at all about the purpose of this visit. Following the standards of work with children in Ukraine, parents are always present during the initial sessions or consultations, which again R seemed unaware of when his mother brought him into treatment.

When asked whether he saw himself as aggressive, R shrugged and responded with "maybe," explaining that he became angry when his mother made him attend his school classes online. To the analysts it appeared that R did not perceive himself as "aggressive" but that he was also aware of having difficult reactions to attending his school yet again online. It appeared from both R's and his mother's perspective that anger and refusal to go to online school began when they were living as refugees in another country. It appeared that for a long time, while trying to obtain housing and documents in a foreign country, R could not attend school and missed much of his academic year.

In addition, it was revealed that until they crossed the borders, R had no idea they were leaving Ukraine as refugees but was continually told that they were traveling as tourists for a leisure trip. Certainly, we recognize that at his age R was aware of the war conditions but had to navigate the escape on his own as a response to mother's minimization and lie. As discussed below, it was far more likely R's response of anger was to this outright falsehood and treatment of him as an object by his mother who needed to act in accordance with her own well-defended position that denied him any space to subjectively experience the things he knew, felt, and saw. Similarly, R had to contend with his subjective knowledge about his step-father's participation on the front lines in Ukraine's military defense against Russian aggression. R then shared that he was very angry that he was not told about his stepfather for a long while and that he was continually worried about him as well as very proud of him.

In that initial session, R's mother was able to acknowledge her fears of sharing difficult information with R, considering him "too small" to understand such things as fleeing as refugees or military service to defend Ukraine. However, this infantilization of R by his mother denied his developmental psychological capacities and his awareness as well as affective reactions as a 10-year-old pre-teen. Mother seemed somewhat aware of the impact of her lies on her child yet did not appear to understand how her infantilized objectification of R denied his subjective reality and denied him space for his own relationship to factual world and experiences.

Another significant concern that emerged during this session was that the mother stressed that she felt overwhelmed and guilty for not ensuring her son continued schooling while they were refugees. While her concerns might be understandable, her defended reaction to her lack as a parent was to return to Ukraine and to drop her son off with her estranged parents. Importantly, R had no relation to his maternal grandparents, having never met them and in fact did not even know their names. The mother did not make it clear to the therapist that her son was not properly acquainted with his grandparents and that she had dropped him off with her parents without any introduction. She was in her profoundly psychotic disassociated state avoiding and running away to work and processing documents for returning to Ukraine, in order to avoid emotional experiences—this did not make it clear that her son was not properly acquainted with his grandparents.

Thus, mother's focus on R's supposed tantrums in response to attending online classes took on entirely different meaning when R was abandoned with no information with people who were total strangers, who were then tasked with ensuring that he now attended school. Lies, omission, abandonment, and accusations, directed at R and supposedly for his benefit, occurred while denying his reality (e.g., "protecting" him from "truth of war," or "making sure he goes to school").

In this session, the mother's need for control, and control beyond typical parental supervision, was palpable. In the session, an interpretation was made that in the circumstances of a war, which cannot be controlled, she grasped for all forms of control, including significantly increased forms of control over her son's life. However, the analyst was also aware and bringing into the session the importance of understanding how such methods of control via defended means that denied R's subjective reality were destructive. Leaving R with estranged and unconnected relatives or threatening to leave him there if he did not comply, were also discussed as problematic. Mother and son agreed to have R stay with her while R still had to negotiate his mother's needs by promising to be more open to online schooling.

In the second session, the mother and the son came together again. R appeared in more positive mood and seemed more talkative but continued to indicate that he did not wish to meet alone with the analyst for any period of time. It was not clear for whom the insistence on joint meeting was made. On one hand, analyst was aware that R was "left" before and as a child would have been anxious to use any such acts as a form of maternal challenges with his separateness, his needs, or his subjective affects, likely reflecting her own struggles with Oedipal processes. On the other hand, it seemed that the mother could not allow her son, who was now old and capable enough, of holding a relational therapeutic space with an analyst on his own subjective terms.

During the session the mother praised R but also continually threatened him that if his "tantrums" and "aggression" returned, he would be again left alone with his grandparents. While R continually assured his mother he would continue to be on his best behavior and wanted to stay with his mother. While it seemed that he developed some relationship with his grandparents (he at least was told their names!), it was clear that he had little to no connection to them outside of his own efforts. R shared attempting a relational bond by initiating activities with them like going to the park.

The session appeared productive. Mother and the son seemed to hold some communication about their needs, and mother showed openness to interpretations and suggestions. However, at the end of the session, when R stepped out to use the bathroom, the mother turned to the analyst demanding to know if the analyst agrees with her that aggressive that his behavior is aggressive. This ending highlighted the continued dissonance between how the other perceived her son's behavior, which was in opposition to realities of the session or the analyst experiences of R. She continued to be unwilling to face her reactions to her son's healthy separateness from her defenses, especially her denial, disassociation, and insistence on maintaining maternal defenses in regard to war, his step-father, his grandparents, or his schooling. The analyst encouraged the mother to return to treatment. The analyst offered to discuss this issue in the next session, because the time of this session had already ended. Despite the mother's assurances, she no-showed for next sessions.

Case Discussion

This case highlights the challenges of parents, as well as patients and analysts, efforts to better regulate strong emotions, whether it is anger, sadness, fear, or anxiety. In the case, presented above, usual interpretations would focus on Oedipal and parental dynamics, on varied aspects of object relatedness, and developmental milestones, which often require children to develop affects and behaviors that come in conflict with parents. In this case, it is also evident that the mother is overwhelmed by her own similar effects of anger, anxiety, sadness, and so forth, which she controls both in her son and via her decisions to pass him on to grandparents. In addition, whether war-related or certainly her own psychology-based (i.e., complete estrangement from her parents), the mother's defensive reality, which is precipitated by severe stress and distress, is activated when she maintains the need to deny reality, to infantilize her son, act profoundly aggressively toward him (e.g., leave him with strangers with no explanation), and disassociation. The mother uses avoidance and escape as defense mechanisms that do not give her the opportunity to accompany her son in the process of growing up. Her projection of her own aggression is evident in this case since any act of separateness of distress by R for truly valid reasons is interpreted as his "aggression" or "tantrums."

In accord with psychoanalytic theories, we believe that R's anger and aggression were important tools in defense of his subjectivity, considering that his life was upended and then managed by others, including his mother. In our view, R's refusal to engage in mother's denials and other defenses was important and healthy, yet as her child he had to navigate the Oedipal, developmentally appropriate and life-based realities: R cannot physically survive without his mother. R's anger toward distancing, abandonment, and detachment were also evident in his case—not only in reactions to his yet-again remote learning but also in violently enforced distance from his home, his step-father, as well as his entire life of childhood friends and activities. Fleeing war violence as refugees is NOT a tourist leisure trip, and R, like all Ukrainian children with capacity for such cognitive awareness, knew this. His distress at both being left behind by his mother or perceptions of being kept away from her is psychically adaptive.

In these circumstances the challenge remains in the analytic maintenance of normalization of anger and as not only appropriate human affective function but as appropriate for responses to war conditions. Certainly, analysts agree that aggression and anger are both biologically and socially human and (importantly) vital for human development and setting of boundaries (Lorenz, 2021). However, the term "aggression," as used in sessions by R's mother, also denotes all manner of human behavior—from sadistic cruelty and militarized violence (as showcased by the Russian authorities and their troops) as well as more normative behaviors such as conflict, negative interactions, child tantrums, self-protective behaviors, and so forth.

Another issue, which we see in this case and encounter in our work when working with Ukrainian children during wartime, is the issue of guilt. The guilt is ever-present in R's life, whether in being forced (under false pretenses) to leave his stepfather and his country or in bringing any challenges to his mother. R must contend with unconscious recognition that his mother is lying to him and infantilizing him for his "own good," and that she herself is struggling to survive the war and its losses, which would further induce his guilt. While most adults in these circumstances experience guilt, children face significantly more challenging conditions in which to express confusing feelings and needs in relation to adults about whom they hold guilt. On the other hand, Ukrainian adults, swept up in the importance of patriotism and resistance to Russian aggression, may have a difficult time realizing that children can feel complex reactions of fear, anger, anxiety, and guilt toward varied aspects of war. In our view, it is truly paramount to create safe therapeutic containers in which Ukrainian children can begin to comfortably express a wide range of their feelings.

Analysts recognize that guilt is a complex human emotion that combines affective experiences of suffering, despondency, and depression together with a sense of helplessness and worry. On the other hand, guilt is among the most vital emotions that can allow human beings to take stock of their actions, wonder about their wrongdoings or mistakes, and struggle with failures to reach the "ideal" behaviors, all of which can lead to healthy individuals toward considering and adapting their ego states and actions. Thus, the feeling of guilt seems to be designed to perform the functions of a moral ego or superego regulator, supporting the fulfillment of prosocial norms. In addition, healthy experiences of guilt are central to influencing the formation of self-attitudes and object relations. Therefore, guilt can play both a constructive and a destructive role in the development of the personality (Ulichnyi, 2021).

In times of war, every person affected will seek to do their part to hasten the victory, even young children. Children, like adults, want to expedite the return of life toward normalcy to ensure its safe course. Thus, children also try to contribute to the end of the war by showing their patriotic feelings through actions, yet we believe it is important for practitioners and parents to recognize that for children, the price of using their guilt in pursuit of social control may be higher than for adults.

Zagorodniuk (2022), in her contribution entitled *Listening to Children through the Experience of War and Mourning,* discussed the experiences of a noted pediatrician and child psychoanalyst, Dolto (2018), who herself survived two global wars. In that description and Dolto's (2023) own accounts, the profound challenges and influence on a child (including knowing early on that she would become a "child doctor") are discussed, including Dotlo's response to her parents when she was a young child, facing a world war: "Children can be bothered by things that are inside and are not germs" (p. 41). Somehow, in words remembered from war-affected childhood, we can find that children are highly sensitive to their contexts of war and that their patriotism and courage are equally bound by their confusion and guilt.

Children and teens can be profoundly overwhelmed by a sense of responsibility and guilt in times of war (Zagorodniuk, 2022). Healthy patriotism, in our view, is also possible among children who can develop it through meaningful identification, rather than guilt. This patriotism appears to grow through identification with their fathers who are serving to defend Ukraine in the military, or parents who volunteer. It often motivates children to join with their parents through child's own subjective experience. We have observed children gain psychic strength and inner satisfaction in possibility of engaging in patriotic actions through their own choices or actions.

In Ukraine, understandably, adults and children are watching news stories about Ukrainian defenders who "lay their lives" for others and the country or who "died so we can live." Many Ukrainian adults in the media share stories of their children raising money, baking or writing letters to Ukrainian defenders. Yet, as psychoanalysts, we also have to recognize that young children and teens experience many profoundly challenging emotions when they are met with such life tasks. Whether in self-psychology or other analytic theories, psychoanalytic literature stresses that children must have space for healthy experiences of narcissism, egocentrism, and self-focus (Chekstere, 2008). In addition, we know from psychoanalytic theories that in a child's mind, adults leave (including to fight war tyrants) not because of adult reasoning but because (children worry) about something they did or did not do.

These are profoundly challenging topics to discuss and consider, including "on the ground" when working with families and children affected by the ongoing war. However, in our opinion, one of the best strategies for parents and other adults is to make space for children to talk about the war by asking them for what they see/feel/experience/observe, including numerous complex emotional reactions. The goal should be to create an open, safe space for children to talk about the war and their perceptions of it without fear or an expectation of a "correct" response.

In our view, our young patient R did express his patriotism through his powerful feelings for his stepfather on the front lines. On the other hand, children like R must be given space for their subjective reality and understanding of war. Lies, denials, minimizations, or gaslighting might be damaging to children while also evoking a response to them. In order to mitigate the abovementioned sense of guilt, children and teens like R could be offered space for their subjective affective realities, their observations, their experiences, and their questions. Parents and other adults must further learn that their own projected guilt via insistence on their child's particular patriotic responses can further foster child's own guilt along with the unbearable burden of their parents' (Zagorodniuk, 2022).

In our opinion, in no way should we devalue the lives that were taken by hiding what was happening from the child. It is important to speak correctly about the war, which can act as a prevention of the emergence of a sense of guilt in children. By the word "correct" we understand that talking with children about the war begins with choosing a time, place and asking the child: "What did you see/hear?", "What do you think?", that is, giving the children the first word. This open inquiry might help adults understand how a child, as a subject of war and life, experiences, feels and perceives the war. In case of R, his subjective reality, his objectification and infantilization, his experiences of war (including his deep care for his step-father on the frontlines), and his resistance to external and intersubjective violence were/will be important to hold in analytic spaces. Using the metaphor of child learning to ride a bike, R's subjective reality is his own bicycle, without which R is given no space to be and become.

Psychoanalysis with Children and Adolescents during the War

Psychoanalysis with children and teens who are in the midst of an active war experience is not well discussed in the field. From our lived direct experiences as child psychoanalysts, we affirm that child analysis is extremely difficult during the wartime, including also because of a high risk to the psychoanalyst's life (e.g., missile attacks), the unstable conditions (e.g., power outages, air raids), the variability of the environment, and often limited access to regular analytic space. The experiences of the invasion, war, and occupation go beyond everyday human experience and leave behind pain, suffering, grief, fear, anxiety, and despair. These potent events leave a scarring imprint on the psyche of children, often rendering traditional methods and strategies of psychoanalysis unattainable in working with them, as we described above. We are continually aware that daily Russian military threats to our lives means that at any time the training wheels (from the metaphor above) can be violently removed from children's bicycles. Death or the threat of death to child's analyst has the capacity to hold profound psychic violence which Ukrainian children carry in relation to fear for lives of their parents, siblings, friends, and others.

Socrates is believed to have said, "Speak so I can see you," but we, as Ukrainian analysts, recognize that we often are unable to see or hear the child in these times. Even if willing, we are physically unable to provide the psychoanalytic safe containers for our young analysands. Thus, psychoanalysis with children becomes nearly impossible during the war for many reasons, including numerous practical barriers such as safety concerns and instability in the lives of parents and analysts. In addition, the formation of transference and countertransference are intersubjectively disrupted and externally influenced. Last, the issue of payment and other aspects of the typical analytic frame also become interrupted, over which children have no control.

The first reason for the unfeasibility of child psychoanalysis in the conditions of war, in our view, is related to parents. Certainly, Ukrainian parents appeal to us as psychoanalysts with urgent requests to help their children, often flooding our phone message lines with such requests. We hear from parents who describe themselves as drowning in despair, powerlessness, fear, and anxiety, which often they connect not to the war itself but to their terror about the child's conditions as the result of war. These parents, who might withstand danger directed at them, struggle to face their children's distress, which they typically do not understand and cannot endure. Parents who reach us tend to describe two types of conditions that significantly worry them about their children: their children's paralyzing anxiety symptoms or their children's expressions of anger, rage, or aggression toward their environment. We hear, over and over, parents say: "I do not recognize my child," "I don't know what to do," "I'm terrified out of my mind," "I can't control/I lose control," and so forth. Among Ukrainian parents of young children, the most prevalent conditions are children's severe anxiety, phobias, enuresis, nightmares, selective mutism, and severe tantrums. Among adolescents, parents call in with concerns about their teens' premature or non-boundaried sexual behavior, isolation, self-harm, panic attacks, depression, suicidality, and so forth.

Certainly, as psychoanalysts, we understand that these extreme behaviors and affective states, among both adults and their children, are the result of the daily confrontation Ukrainians experience with death and the risk of death. All of these Ukrainians have faced unspeakable terror and losses, yet in addition majority of them also face additional realities of grief in losing relatives and friends, witnessing torture and destruction of people they know, and encounters with intense traumatizing events. In our view, and that of our colleagues (Nalyvaiko, 2023), the most common affective challenge for Ukrainian children (and adults) is related to varied forms of severe anxiety.

Particularly, as we name numerous and varied concerns, there is one shared context of these challenges—the war. Many parents and other adult caregivers react to this war context and its inhuman impact on psychic lives with significant regression. Dorozhkin (2023) repeatedly noted the state of regression under war conditions among adults. At times, when we communicate with parents, it was not their children who required therapeutic containment but the parents themselves. Often, we had to respond with active supportive, grounding, and psychoeducational material for the parent, which at times seemed all that was needed so that the parent could (temporarily) find their ego resources to continue their lives and parenting roles. At times, we knew that parent hid their children, typically unconsciously, from us as analysts, or rather, they seemed unable or fearful of having their children bring their own subjectivity and needs into an analytic space.

As we write this, we are aware of stories of Ukrainian parents we know and worked with who literally had to save themselves and their children by hiding out in cellars or basements, covering their children's mouths to remain quiet so that the Russian soldiers would not find them. All Ukrainians in Russian-occupied territories witnessed how often families and children could be taken, tortured, or executed right in front of parents as Russians sought to violently impose their control upon these Ukrainian areas. In some ways, even after the threats to life have passed, it seems like Ukrainian parents struggle to let their children "make sounds" or speak about their experience lest they may be once again "found and killed." War is the kind of Real, which Lacan (2014) described in his work about anxiety as an encounter with the Real. The subject disappears, and the anxiety in the face of the terrifying Real can become overwhelming. Such a response is also biologically understandable for numerous living species. Certainly, in Ukraine, as a country that continues to experience daily Russian military attacks, these reactions are understandable.

The second reason for the impossibility of starting and continuing child analysis during the war is related to the analysts themselves. Children's analysts in Ukraine, from the first days, were also directly touched on the horrors of war. Every feeling experienced by both the young patients and their parents was something that the analysts have felt: fear, uncertainty, loss of control, and rage were what most, if not all, Ukrainians felt. The peculiarity of these feelings is that, first, they have a significant intensity, and second, that they resonate with the patients' affective states. Analysts in the process of analysis are tasked with containing what is unbearable for their own patients, yet in this case they all must hold these experiences for themselves also. We have recognized that such double containerization oversaturates the psyche and causes fatigue, exhaustion, and burnout among Ukrainian psychoanalysts. Certainly, as psychoanalysts, we do have our own analysis and supervision, which help to withstand this mental load. Thus, typically, most of us show up for our patients because we rely on some containment for ourselves but also because we know we must.

Therefore, the formation of transference and countertransference reactions, central to the psychoanalytic process, becomes complicated. On one hand, the analyst's office must contain the violence or anxiety that is not just psychic but literal and real when the Other seeks to destroy you and your patients via varied means of war. We also see that parents fear, unconsciously, that the rage and anger, held by their children, could be directed at them or us the analysts, worrying that it might harm the adults.

The final obstacle to starting or continuing child analysis, which we wish to highlight here, is related to payment as part of the therapeutic frame. As analysts and citizens, we cannot ignore the really difficult economic situation in Ukraine since so many individuals have lost access to any form of financial support. However, for both the analysts and the parents, not paying directly limits long-term possibilities for psychoanalytic services. Therefore, many Ukrainian citizens turn toward free help or services for minimal payment, which tends to be crisis-oriented and limited in time.

Unfortunately we as analysts cannot work only pro-bono when our livelihood is dependent on payment for our services (e.g., Ukraine does not have external insurance payment schemes common in other countries). Moreover, from Freud's works, also occurring during the times of war and lack, we recognize that payment for services and the exchange of money is central to the formation of the therapeutic frame and the intersubjective containment (Hart & Linda Jacobsen, 2019; Kaplin et al., 2019). Many parents we work with understand that quick crisis care, which is free, cannot replace more in-depth and individualized care for their children. For many parents, on the other hand, money also becomes a symptom of their regression: they wish for their analysts to become all-loving parents who would sacrifice themselves for their children without asking for anything in return.

In addition, the difficult work of being with children who are affected by war (and their parents) is that it takes tremendously longer at times to establish trust, to ensure the therapeutic alliance and container, to work through screen symptoms, to foster space in which defenses (including regression) can be experienced and held, and to allow for working through. We continually witness the exhaustion and the impossibility of being parents under conditions of war and see how payment is often one aspect of this struggle. In initial consultations with parents' money is often a signifier of many other aspects of parents' lives.

Conclusion

In this contribution, we highlight that in a metaphor of child as learning to ride a bicycle by not only having an access to their own subjective experience but also to "training wheels" support of parents and analysts, among others, highlights that war conditions are the attack on the entirety of this experience. As we noted in case of R, war exacerbates problems, and with compromised access to psychoanalytic care, further exacerbates challenges for children to find analytic containment or support. The entire bicycle is at risk of literally being violently destroyed. Moreover, children must learn to "ride" in such conditions while holding experiences of guilt, aggression, anxiety, and grief. Certainly, in ordinary times and healthy circumstances children's lives, including children who have faced challenges, both parents and analysts serve as such wheels of care and support.

We end our contribution with a special thank you to Dr. Carol Fahy, who supported our work by hearing us analytically and bringing together our thoughts toward a metaphor. As we continue to work in Ukraine under conditions of Russian war violence we continue to explore ways to understand and respond to what happens between parents, children, and analysts during the war.

We express our gratitude to Dr. Oleksandr Lupis for editorial contribution and assistance in conveying our experience in the text

References

Chekstere, O. Y. (2008). Views of J. Piaget on the peculiarities of egocentrism of children's thinking. *Actual Problems of Psychology: Psychology of Learning. Genetic Psychology. Medical Psychology*, 10, 32–42.

Dolto, F. (2018). *Fighting for a child.* Family Leisure Club.

Dolto, F. (2023). *On the child's side.* Center for Educational Literature.

Dorozhkin, V. (2023). Modern warfare and its impact on the therapeutic relationship. *Ukrainian Psychoanalytic Journal*, 1(1), 32–35. https://doi.org/10.32782/upj/2023-1-6

Hart, S., & Linda Jacobsen, S. (2019). The emotional development scale: Assessing the emotional capacity of 4–12 years olds. *Journal of Infant, Child, and Adolescent Psychotherapy*, 18(2), 185–195.

Kaplin, D., Parente, K. & Santacroce, F. A. (2019). A review of the use of trauma systems therapy that treat refugee children, adolescents, and families. *Journal of Infant, Child, and Adolescent Psychotherapy*, 18(4), 417–431.

Lacan, J. (2014). The mirror stage as formative of the function of the I as revealed in psychoanalytic experience. In *Reading French Psychoanalysis*. Routledge.

Lorenz, K. (2021). *On aggression*. Routledge.

Nalyvaiko, N. (2023). Linguistic metamorphoses as representations of subjectivity. Ukraine. War diary. *Ukrainian Psychoanalytic Journal*, 1, 27–31. https://doi.org/10.32782/upj/2023-1-5

Ulichnyi, I. L. (2021) The main functions of the manifestation of guilt. *5th International scientific and practical conference "European scientific discussions"* (March 28–30, 2021), 453.

Zagorodniuk, N. (2022). Listening to children through the experience of war and mourning. *Fragments of the speech at the 4th scientific and practical all-Ukrainian conference "Psychoanalysis. Revisiting by the war. Ethics, clinic and personal experience"*, October 22–23, 2022. Kyiv.

Chapter 13

Wartime Supervision as Psychoanalytical Research of Clinical Cases and Psychic Phenomena

Volodymyr Mamko

The Psychoanalytic Approach and Supervision in Crisis Work

Certain aspects of supervising psychoanalytic therapy during wartime are specific and unique. Supervision is expected to effectively assist in addressing many complex and conflicting issues, urgent and relevant. By the start of the war, we already had experience organizing and conducting therapeutic work and supervision in extraordinary conditions. This experience is owed to our recent political and professional history.

We began our activities back in 2009. Since then, we have worked in crisis psychology based on a psychoanalytic approach. This means that we utilized psychoanalytic theory (Freud, Klein, Bion, Lacan, and others), psychoanalytic technical approaches (of course, the concept of the psychoanalytic setting, therapeutic alliance), and consistently worked with the analysis of transference and resistance. Accordingly, supervision of crisis work was also conducted based on the psychoanalytic approach to training, practice control, and working with complex cases. This approach allowed us to provide a comprehensive view of our psychoanalytic, therapeutic, and crisis practice.

Supervision has become fundamental to the organizational structure of crisis assistance. Supervision was mandatory, intensive, and frequent. For example, for every three hours of work with victims and those who have experienced severe trauma, at least one hour of supervision was provided. If work was carried out for many hours a day or over several days, supervisors themselves also had to undergo supervision. Thus, supervision was placed at the core of psychological assistance as a mandatory and central element of the entire complex of crisis response measures. At the organizational level, it prioritized and ensured the achievement of goals and tasks of the

DOI: 10.4324/9781032660257-14

whole system of psychological assistance. We can attest that supervision effectively provided prevention and prophylaxis of professional burnout and secondary psychological traumatization. Direct participants of supervision groups and their close circle, including relatives, colleagues, friends, unequivocally benefited from the positive effects.

It is important to emphasize that our methodology of applying supervision in training crisis psychology has proven very positive as a method of education and professional training. After theoretical training in the fundamentals of crisis psychology and practical work with victims (i.e., patients), novice therapists gained their first experience reviewing their actions as psychoanalytic therapists in educational supervision. We conducted extensive crisis, therapeutic, and academic work during the period of civil unrest in Kyiv in 2013–2014 and military actions in southeastern Ukraine in 2014–2016. This work helped numerous analysts acquire particular professional experience. Additionally, dozens of our current colleagues were able to start their practice during that period and subsequently thrive in their profession.

Such previous experience immensely helped us to respond to the onset of military actions in 2022 promptly, the evacuation and resettlement of around 10 million residents of Ukraine, and the mass extermination of the civilian population. We needed to immediately conduct express training on the basics of crisis assistance, determine the order and modes of operation of crisis groups, and most importantly, establish and ensure continuous operation of a supervisory project to ensure the safety of working psychoanalysts, psychotherapists, and consultants.

Therefore, we immediately started the crisis assistance project named "War Time Research." The project began on March 3, 2022, and has been ongoing. Participants in our groups always have the opportunity to seek and receive supervisory support both in group settings and individually. Our project has at least seven group supervisions conducted per week. Over the past year, the project has benefited from continuous collaboration with colleagues from the Eyra Psychosocial Assistance organization (Massachusetts, USA), who conduct at least two weekly group supervisions. This project is supported by the resources of the Institute of Professional Supervision (Kyiv, Ukraine).

The primary goal was to implement the critical principle of crisis assistance: to ensure the safety and functionality of the helping practice. Without this, the hope for deploying an emergency infrastructure, whose task should be: (1) to ensure and support the stability of the previous practice, i.e., the one that was functioning before the war, and (2) to deploy a working regime in conditions of an extraordinary crisis – war – disappears.

It can be said that at the very beginning, our goal was not solely a supervisory project. Initially, it was a virtual refuge where one could seek shelter from uncertainty and upheavals to provide mental health professionals with the required support, as McWilliams (2023) emphasized. The refuge was primarily intended for psychoanalysts, psychotherapists, and clinical psychologists. The reader may benefit from the report of one of this project participants – Elina Yevlanova (2023) – who described this experience both as supervision and self-care valuable in wartime. However, we understood that we could not and should not restrict access to anyone. Therefore, at the initial stage, for the first two to four months, it was completely open and available to all individuals seeking psychological help.

The Influence of Supervision on the Training and Development of Analysts in Wartime

During the most challenging initial period, participants in our groups often expressed the need to receive clarification on various issues. It appeared that by the start of supervision, none of the participants had a clinical case report for some reason. However, there was a need to understand how to act or interpret certain aspects of psychoanalytic theory in the applied clinical field. This need to verbalize their experience was expressed as a question to the supervisor, formulated in a more or less reasoned manner. Clarifying the question and providing a rational explanation was generally well-received and usually led to constructive and friendly discussions. The participants' need for an open and honest supervisor appears evident. Engaging in joint research of professional issues or clinical case circumstances involves successful and erroneous decisions and reflections.

Allowing oneself and others such a degree of freedom can be instructive. In the context of challenging military and clinical circumstances, it is essential to learn to overcome not only internal representations of hierarchical limitations and power dynamics of more experienced and knowledgeable colleagues and mentors but also to demonstrate that there is nothing shameful in not only acknowledging one's lack of knowledge but also admitting one's mistakes. It is also crucial to affirm that even having a firmly grounded professional position regarding a clinical case does not preclude insisting on one's particular assessment and conducting further case exploration, maintaining the possibility of discovering one's way to verify the truth or falsehood of the chosen strategy.

As experience shows, little can compare in value to learning from one's experience; moreover, when the conditions of such learning are provided in the form of a collective charged with honest work and dedicated to their profession, attentive mentors, and an awareness of their essential mission for their patients. Unfortunately, the lack of opportunity for psychotherapists to participate in supervision projects during wartime or the refusal to engage in such projects under intense, "worn-out" conditions of work in the harsh conditions of war leads to the effect that after some time, therapists who do not undergo supervision appear less confident than before. Supervisory control indicates that their professional skill has also decreased, often quite drastically. From this position, it can be concluded that for professional well-being and development, personal work experience alone is not sufficient. Without constant and intensive supervision and analytical processing of one's experience, the mistakes to which a therapist is usually prone only intensify. This is especially true considering such work is carried out in unfamiliar, volatile, and often dangerous conditions.

It must be acknowledged that errors in work are exacerbated because the therapist's previous psychoanalytic training was insufficiently thorough and of poor quality upon closer examination – something we all regret belatedly. However, there is a positive aspect: many things become clear. Now, retrospectively, we can critically observe many elements of our previous professional and student experience and personal analysis. The humility of the supervisees, with which they accept that their past was not only imperfect but sometimes outright wrong, is sometimes astonishing. Such an open and restrained attitude towards their recent persistence in erroneous approaches, as well as acknowledging their committed and already, unfortunately, irreparable mistakes, is evidence of significant professional and personal growth of the therapist. This position contributes to the fact that some psychoanalysts in our project consider undergoing a repeat experience of personal analysis or treatment. The fact that such a desire arises due to a two-year, very intensive training project indicates that exploring one's unconscious becomes an urgent need for the therapist, even in the most challenging life circumstances.

It is important to note that the strategy in which the supervisor consistently takes an openly active and supportive position during work, in our view, has proven itself. The entire organization and conduct of supervision, starting from a very reliable setting and internal rules, including the supervisor's devotion and stability, as far as possible, compensated for the lack of stability and security in the world surrounding the psychotherapeutic space. Besides the opportunity to identify with an external reliable figure or object, this strategy allows for resorting to defensive projection, thereby sharing responsibility with this reliable figure for possible mistakes and missteps.

The therapeutic setting underwent significant changes with the onset of war. It changed suddenly and irreversibly. Military actions and the wave of evacuations led to the cessation of therapy due to the rupture of therapeutic bonds. Initially, almost all therapy sessions were canceled from the first hours of the war. Most sessions were canceled without prior notice or warning. The payment arrangements for sessions were also completely disrupted if they were not paid for individually. There were widespread ruptures and terminations of therapeutic relationships. This happened abruptly, massively, with half-words, and irreversibly. Only now can we remember some of the patients whom their therapists forgot. Similarly, therapists found themselves abandoned and lost by their patients. Typically, only those pairs who shared the conditions of their existence remained. For example, both participants of the therapeutic pair stayed in Ukraine or, conversely, left the country and started a vastly different life as refugees and emigrants. Those who could share similarity and stability in their external context relative to their therapeutic relationships survived. Thus, the observations lead us to conclude that the setting should be associated with strength and stability – the representability – of each other's perceptions. Conversely, the lack of descriptive reality or presumed awareness of the patient about the therapist's living conditions hinders the continuation of the analysis. Such impossibility eliminates the basis of transference and the therapeutic alliance. Swift and unpredictable changes in a patient's life, the variety of events, and the intensity of impressions lead the person in therapy to try to rid themselves of therapeutic relationships as untimely, out-of-phase, incongruent, and alien objects. Therapy acts as a tightly laced corset of the setting, artificially stable and inhibited by external efforts. Perhaps the strict setting functions as a means of enhancing the functions of the Superego, thereby strengthening the Ego as a whole (Freud, 1926). This contributes to rigidity towards impulses of the Id, events, and impressions of external reality. Such limited mobility leads to a restriction in the use of psychic resources and, consequently, to its traumatization. In the absence of compensatory and corrective interventions by the therapist, the patient resorts to acting out and interrupting therapy. This absence occurs due to the therapist's inability to intervene and soften the patient's harsh Superego, which criticizes and inhibits the Ego flooded with Id impulses. In transference, this structural conflict is extrapolated onto the therapist.

The absence of the necessary support in terms of a reliable setting and required intervention from the therapist leads to the rupture of therapeutic relationships. This expresses the impossibility of existing under the yoke of circumstances of irresistible force. The acting out of escaping from occupation also occurs when the civilian setting of peacetime is replaced by the unregulated "as if" setting of wartime. Readiness for exploration and corresponding changes is a characteristic feature of analytical work in wartime.

Studying Trauma Therapy in Supervision

Supervisee – a Ukrainian female, who is a refugee, psychotherapist working in a psychodynamic approach, specializing in working with children and adolescents, university professor, and regular participant in the supervision project. The presented case of supervision is published with her consent, while case content was disguised for confidentiality purposes.

Case Presentation

Patient: 8-year-old child, boy, Ukrainian, status – a military refugee granted temporary protection in a European country. The family consists of a mother, father, and child. The family arrived in the host country in May 2022. The child started first grade in the same year. Previously, the family lived in Mariupol. They came here through Russia. In Russia, they passed through a filtration camp for refugees from Ukrainian territory.

The mother shared the following events and circumstances their family endured. The Russian army's siege of the city was perilous, and evacuation was impossible. For two months, the family lived in the basement of a multi-story building, where about 60 people were staying. Once, in a supermarket, in a fight over the remaining food, one man beat another man to death with a hammer. The boy was with his mother and saw all of this. At another time, the mother bought 2 kg (4.5 lb) of candy for $100 as the only available food. The mother fed the child sparingly with candy. However, other people stole their candy at night. The child knew and saw all of this. They witnessed the death of their neighbor from artillery shelling. The man was left without a face. He ran and helped others for some time and then died at the basement door. The child saw this.

There were cases when people living in the basement did not let newly arrived people seek shelter. She mentions this and recalls a woman with a child. But the mother managed to defend a wounded German shepherd that wandered in. She treated it and left it in the basement.

None of the women in the cellar agreed to cook food on the fire outside. Only the boy's mother went out to do it. That same shepherd heard mortar shots that people couldn't hear and, howling, ran into the basement first. The mother ran after the dog. Behind her, the blasts of incoming shells rang out. Shrapnel from the shells rattled against the iron door of the basement.

The mother treated the wounds of many people. She estimates that she helped around 80 people. She bandaged wounds, gave injections, and nursed civilians and military personnel. Then, she transferred them to military units and other places for further care.

She helped 130 dogs and cats abandoned by their owners. She saved them, persuaded people to take them under their care, or handed them to someone to look after. The mother slept little and almost always ran out of the basement to help, leaving the child alone in his sleeping place.

In Mariupol, "the dead started coming to her in her sleep" (quote). She knew their names and other details. The next day, she would find on social networks that someone was looking for these people. These predictive dreams scared her. She was afraid to talk to anyone about it and was equally scared to sleep.

The mother brought the boy to therapy by referral from the school and a diagnostic center where the school psychologist referred him.

The child is restless and emotionally torn. The child has shown multiple symptoms of post-traumatic stress disorder. He experiences frequent outbursts and depressive symptoms, displays avoidant behavior, lacks positive emotions, has become less active, and even refuses his favorite activities. For example, he refuses to eat regular food like beet soup (borscht) because it is "too red." He also has extreme intolerance and sensitivity to sharp and loud sounds. He panics, covers his ears, starts crying, and has difficulty stopping. They tried to help him at school by giving him headphones to reduce his reaction to sounds. The recommendations of psychologists are almost impossible to follow due to the language barrier and the lack of qualified specialists for such a severe disorder.

The child is easy to engage with and talks willingly but does not expect any response in return. Moreover, he tends to ignore speech directed at him, saying, "I don't trust anyone here" (quote). In Ukraine, he had many friends whom he trusted. He interacts with many people, but in reality, he trusts no one. He experiences flashbacks that lead him to states where he loses control. When in such a state, he "disappears." He often has nightmares. According to his mother, they had a pet cat in the family. During the shelling of Mariupol, the cat was hit and died from multiple shrapnel wounds. The mother intentionally did not tell her son about this, saying the cat ran away from home. The boy constantly carries a toy that looks like a live cat but has glass eyes. This cat is always with him.

Traumatic dream. Every night, he dreams of his cat. The boy says, "At first, she is affectionate, rubbing against my legs. Then she suddenly attacks me. Scratching my legs, biting, there is blood, flesh, bones. Then my mom appears. She has a big knife in her hands." She protects the boy, attacking the cat. "One-two, and – zero!" – the boy expressively comments on the action and its result. When asked about the meaning of his words, he cannot say anything coherent.

Language situation. Although the child's parents come from the traditionally Russian-speaking east of Ukraine, and the family has always lived in that Russian-speaking region (a large industrial center on the shore of the Sea of Azov – the city of Mariupol, probably the most destroyed and affected by the war among other Ukrainian towns), currently the mother and the child speak exclusively Ukrainian. The father can also speak Ukrainian now but can effortlessly switch to Russian and speak it. The child cannot maintain a conversation in Russian. When spoken to in Russian, he stops understanding the speech directed at him and almost immediately loses the ability to focus on and understand it; "everything falls apart and disappears" (quote). The local educational system and psychological services cannot give proper attention to children in Ukrainian or Russian.

Their home in Mariupol is now destroyed, and they have nowhere to return to. In Mariupol, the boy's grandmother and grandfather – his mother's parents – remained. The Russian authorities did not allow them to leave Mariupol and enter Russian territory. The boy's family went through a filtration camp.

Recently the grandfather passed away. The boy's mother could not attend the funeral in Mariupol. Allegedly, the mandatory condition for her entry into that territory was to accept Russian citizenship. As of today, the grandmother is also in feeble health. The mother and grandmother communicate via the Internet several times daily. According to the mother, the grandmother is also in an unsatisfactory psychological state.

The father's brother is in the Armed Forces, on the front line. However, he has been out of contact since January 30. The military enlistment office has issued a certificate stating that he is missing. The father is deeply involved in the search for his brother. He looks exhausted, responds in monosyllables, and appears distracted. The father seems emotionally restrained and closed off. He looks at his wife and child with a unique sense of compassion. He has not shown any initiative or responsiveness toward the therapist or regarding the mental state of the child and wife. He works two jobs to support the family.

Every three sessions with the child, there is one session with the parents, usually only with the mother, as the father is very busy. The mother is worried about the child. However, she always looks tearful and mentally exhausted.

Request to the supervisor: What should I do with them? I got involved in this story with the child. But if the mother were better, I could probably help the child. The mother brings this child to me as if she is pushing the child out of the water onto the shore, as if saying, "Do something with him, at least!" But the child is deteriorating much faster than he is recovering. I wouldn't know that our sessions are without results.

Supervisor: "What does it mean that he is deteriorating faster than he is recovering?"

Some symptoms disappear, while others appear. At least after our sessions, he stopped wearing headphones at school. He can now tolerate sharp sounds much better. But other troubling symptoms have appeared: he asks his mother to paint his nails with nail polish and to put on a girl's dress. Supervisor: "So, there is a change in symptoms?"

Supervisee: Yes. The nightmares have also disappeared. I can't describe the mother as sexual. She seems to represent a particular type of caring for everyone and everything. Like Mother Teresa – she will feed everyone, heal everyone, save all the dogs, and comfort everyone's soul. I can't do classical psychoanalytic work in any form. I have almost come to terms with this. I must disrupt the setting to work with the mother and child simultaneously.

Supervisor: "What do you mean by that?"

When I work with the child, I use parent sessions to shade and explain some competencies to the parent.

Supervisor: "What should such a setting provide in this case? What is its importance? What is its function? I suggest trying to make sense of this now. It may seem too complex or abstract, but we are not in an exam. This is a practical task."

I have my internal barrier. If I overcome it, I am afraid and feel like flying beyond it, as if stepping over my interior setting. I hold onto it as the last thing I have left. Yes, it seems like I am talking about these patients right now. These people seem to be falling. They are very, very traumatized. I try to hold them, detain them, but they still fall. And if I break my setting, I will fall, too. It's like some joint fall that cannot be stopped… With this setting, I have established a fence to hold onto it and say that we have at least saved psychoanalysis.

Supervisor: "What did you mean by the word 'psychoanalysis'?"

Supervisee: You know, it seems to me that this case is not only or primarily a crisis. It feels like there is so much encrypted in it, so much that escapes, that I highly doubt I can limit myself to just crisis work, some affirmations, beliefs, or support of individual mental functions or defenses. Their father acts as a solid support. And I feel furious; I am angry at their father, who remains silent and seems to serve as their support but fails in this mission: he doesn't ask for help himself, doesn't say anything, doesn't respond to anything.

Supervisor: "So, if we rely on the setting, holding on tightly to the setting, but this leads to the failure and downfall of everyone: the boy, the mother, the father, the analyst, … and even psychoanalysis?! You need help. In countertransference, you feel like a support that is not coping with the presented task."

Supervisee: Yes, I feel this way: I feel like the last support and stronghold. This is how the school, diagnostic organization, and everyone else see me, too!

Supervisor: "I draw your attention to the fact that you now state that you critically need help. I remind you of the fundamental principle and the first rule of crisis intervention: the basis of crisis work is to ensure the safety and well-being of the helping psychologist."

Supervisor's intervention: You are the one who protects but can no longer protect. You cannot bear a particular burden, yet you cannot break it

> down. It's as if you are doomed to confrontation and protection. Something needs to be protected. And it turns out that you must save a specific setting. I would advise you not to separate the mother and child in sessions. Let them be in sessions together. You say that the mother does not talk to the child about the death of the cat. Each family member seems locked in a separate speech and language chamber. They are locked in prison chambers of speech and language not assigned to them. In a language not their own, in a language foreign to them, remaining outside the mother's tongue. This disconnection, division, isolation, and fragmentation in speech create a situation where experience is conserved. This protection resists the integration of experience into the Self. Experience must be locked in memories. Memories are separated from speech so that experience does not come alive (Freud, 1899). Of course, déjà vu and repression mechanisms can be rationally explained and even proven. But this distances us from the possibility of making a psychoanalytic interpretation.

We need to figure out how to organize the analytical space better so that there is the possibility of making an analytical interpretation and getting to the very core of the unconscious conflict that triggers the mechanism of symptom formation. What this woman (Mother Teresa) produces is death. Her dreams indicate to us that the object of her desire is death. Her dreams fulfill her desire to see the deceased, help them, and put them to rest.

Direct recommendation: It seems better not to separate the mother and child. You must inquire about this occasionally until the child asks for it himself. And if suggesting it, do so extremely subtly. Right now, however, providing a setting that will allow him to recreate a space in which symbolization can occur, such as the replacement and compensation of memories and impressions through speech, is crucial.

He needs access through maternal language to his mother's body and mother tongue (Dolto, 1984). They regress to the level of preverbal, literal satisfactions. For example, when the boy asks to have his nails painted and to wear a girl's dress, it means that he is experiencing a regression of individual development to the level of gender differentiation (2.5–3 years old). He returns to that age's challenges and begins reliving that stage.

When it comes to what you call multiplication (increasing the quantity and variety) of symptoms, perhaps you should not resist this, not worry about it, not try to oppose it, restrain and suppress this multiplication of symptoms, but instead allow this process to unfold and happen. But this mustn't happen at the expense of your resources because it forces you to experience the patient's conflict directly and react to it with resistance. This should be done through the setting, which should be reliable and appropriate to the possibilities and conditions of clinical work. It would be best if you did not keep the patient on the surface, but the setting should help you with this. Changes in the setting may consist of allowing verbal interaction between mother and child. This is the natural situation where the mother contributes to her child's survival. That is, she deals with death in the name of life – for the survival of her child. Try to rely on the setting and trust the setting. This means trusting your unconscious, as well as depending on theirs. Then, they can reflect and see each other and themselves in a mirror. In this space, they can relate to their shared memories so that a common speech space emerges. The analyst, describing his countertransference, seems to represent a catastrophe happening with patients. They are dying. Without speech, they are drowning. Unable to start speaking, they suffocate.

And also, the cat must die! The toy is the ghost, the specter of the cat. It is also the unburied corpse of a beloved creature. It is a transitional object in regression. Yes, it can be said that this is a transitional object, according to Winnicott (1953). However, it is an object in the transition space, in the space of reciprocal transformation of subject and object. Figuratively, it can be defined as a transitional object between the world of the dead and the living. It remains an open portal, a trace of loss in the self, a witness to depression (Freud, 1917). The cat needs to be buried and mourned. It can be added that the function of the transitional object in this status is a deceased but unburied father. A father who has not undergone a change in his status and has not become a symbolic father. It is the father's corpse that the psychotic left unburied and placed in his house.

These people cannot move on to processing trauma. The trauma remains unhealed and continues to disturb. They are stuck in it. Note that the child develops various metonymic symptoms that do not transition to the level of metaphor. The deficit of repression function is becoming more pronounced (Freud, 1915). The boy experiences a repression failure each time, which he tries to compensate for with denial, splitting, isolation, and abreaction. The mother functions mentally in a similar way. In her dreams, dead people constantly come to her. She cannot bury them. Anxiety is not closed by a symbol. The portal to the infernal space remains open. Dad, mom, and son cannot start talking about murder and death. Beginning to talk about murder means beginning to fit into the symbolic order (Lacan, 1953). Instead, there is identification with the victims, with the missing, with the victims. All members of this family need to be taken out of there, from Mariupol, filled with dead people. "Let the dead bury their dead" Matthew 8:22 (Bible). It is necessary to leave a memorial for the deceased instead of saving them by dragging them away from the grave. Mom usually acts as a resuscitator. Essentially, she denies death with her actions. "They cover up the death, hide it, fragment messages about it, smear it" (supervisee addition).

In sand therapy, a boy shows graves. It is necessary to make graves, funerals, corpses, and dying become the subject of thinking, reminiscing, verbalized impressions, and experiencing the fact of someone's death. It is necessary to strive for them to be capable of spontaneously saying the phrase: "Someone died." This will be a statement, an acknowledgment of the irreversibility of death. "Do you think your cat is alive or already dead? What if she died?" or "Is this a grave? Or is it not a grave? What is a grave? Whose grave is this? How did he die?" – such questions will help the patient rely on the speech of the psychoanalyst.

It seems that the analyst falls into the trap of deceptive obviousness. As if such self-deception frees us from the need to signify, symbolize, and interpret. What is presented, what seems evident without additional words but remains unnamed, actually remains unsymbolized and, accordingly, not integrated, not appropriated. The child invests his affect in form (small mounds of graves), in an object (toy), in a thing (girl's dress), in the body (painted nails), in movement (covering ears), in action (scream, cry), in symptom (request to dress him as a girl), in the dreamlike image (traumatic dream about an attacking cat). However, he does not know how to control, manage, or use them voluntarily. It is necessary to strive to ensure that the setting in therapy helps the psychoanalytic process compensate for the structural elements of the psyche that the patient is deficient in. In the work, it is essential to actively engage patients in this exploration process, carefully monitoring their reactions and interactions with the setting and any attempts to intervene by influencing and changing it. It is important to remember that the setting serves as a space for producing interpretation.

References

Dolto, F. (1984). *L'image inconsciente du corps*. Edition du Seuil.

Freud, S. (1899). Screen memories. *The standard edition of the complete psychological works of Sigmund Freud*. Vol. 20. Translated from German by J. Strachey. London: Hogart Press.

Freud, S. (1915). Repression. *The standard edition of the complete psychological works of Sigmund Freud.* Vol. 14. Translated from German by J. Strachey. London: Hogart Press.

Freud, S. (1917). Mourning and melancholia. *The standard edition of the complete psychological works of Sigmund Freud.* Vol. 14. Translated from German by J. Strachey. London: Hogart Press.

Freud, S. (1926). Inhibitions, symptoms, and anxiety. *The standard edition of the complete psychological works of Sigmund Freud.* Vol. 20. Translated from German by J. Strachey. London: Hogart Press.

Lacan, J. (1953). Fonction et champ de la parole et du langage en psychanalyse. In J. Lacan (Ed.), *Ecrits* (pp. 25–38). AFI.

McWilliams, N. (2023). For my Ukrainian colleagues on a painful anniversary: Some heartful ideas for maintaining practice under fire. *Ukrainian Psychoanalytic Journal*, 1(1), 7–13. https://doi.org/10.32782/upj/2023-1-2

Winnicott, D.W. (1953). Transitional objects and transitional phenomena. *International Journal of Psycho-Analysis*, 34, 89–97.

Yevlanova, E. (2023). Professional supervision as therapists' self-care during wartime. *Psychoanalytic Psychology*, 40(4), 257–260. https://doi.org/10.1037/pap0000486

Chapter 14

He. She. War

Transforming War-Related Experience Through the Intervision Group Dynamics

Veronika Lukyanova and Ruslana Rudenko

Introduction

The war brought an onslaught of emotions—lack of safety, confusion, helplessness, and terror—which prompted a quest for symbolic protection for all influenced by war. To create a safe space in such a time, we (the authors) decided to revive Intervision group meetings with psychologists who were aiding war trauma survivors. The Intervision groups, first introduced and now broadly utilized in the UK and across the world, are non-leader facilitated peer review supervision groups that rely on relational principles and processes to help mental health practitioners deepen their practice, especially in working with trauma (Staempfli & Fairtlough, 2019). We first created an Intervision group for mental health practitioners who were involved in the provision of therapeutic care to civilian and military individuals and families who faced the Russian war in Eastern Ukraine (2014–2018). In February 2022, after a full-scale invasion by the Russian Federation, we re-engaged the group, inviting all practitioners who immediately volunteered to support members of Ukrainian defense forces and their families to participate in a supervision group. We named this group "Vin. Vona. Viyna" (Ukrainian for "He. She. War"). In our name, we wanted to stress not only the fact that both Ukrainian women and men served in the Ukrainian armed forces, defending the country, but also that people of both genders also volunteered or remained behind the frontlines in the care of families.

Psychoanalysts "Just Like the Brothers in Arms"

We first met in Odesa during the summer of 2014 at a German Center—which also served as a local Lutheran church. This location became the home of the Volunteer Psychological Service Odesa, which was founded by the Ukrainian

DOI: 10.4324/9781032660257-15

psychoanalyst Mykhaylo Pustovoyt, who continued to provide psychological support by applying psychoanalytic knowledge to the participants of the Kyiv and Odesa-based Maidan events (Pustovoyt, 2023). For readers not familiar with Maidan events and their vital importance in recent Ukrainian history, Maidan was a form of resistance to pro-Russian political totalitarianism seeking to take over the country in the early 2010s. This organization also began to engage in the terrible aftermath of the Russian invasion, annexation, military actions in the East, and other forms of aggression toward millions of Ukrainians. The volunteer organization was a grassroots effort by the Ukrainian mental health community to aid those who were grappling with the aftermath of the Russian invasion. The project utilized both direct clinical work and also offered two Intervision groups and individual supervision. The first group worked with internally displaced persons (IDPs; millions of Ukrainians lost their homes and became internally displaced after initial Russian occupational attempts in 2014). The second group included clinicians who worked with Ukrainian soldiers and their families. Notably, we were part of the 11-person group working with military members and their families, with all of us notably trained in or drawing on psychoanalytic theories. In contrast, the IDP group of clinicians predominately drew on gestalt and cognitive-behavioral therapy orientations.

Our group focus was on providing peer-based supervision support for those of us who, as clinicians, volunteered our clinical work with active duty military individuals, including providing pro-bono work in military hospitals, rehabilitation programs, and via our own private consulting rooms. We met weekly in the Intervision supervision format while many of us also received and offered supervision elsewhere for this work.

This initial group, created a decade ago, was occurring when war in Ukraine was not as universally experienced as a full-scale invasion. At the time, Russian military actions and Ukrainian defense against them were little recognized worldwide. Work with military members was not popular, including among many psychoanalysts. For many, supporting soldiers was considered a form of supporting the war itself, while many in the psychoanalytic and global community at large just wanted the war to stop. Even in Ukraine, not many individuals fully understood the nature of Russian militarized plans and the nature of their war against Ukraine. Ukrainians have not yet perceived the aggressor nation, which viewed Ukraine as its enemy. Many Ukrainians, despite events of the Maidan revolutions and other liberation independence movements, still have not formed their cultural identity.

Thus, in contrast to the dynamics inside Ukraine and the psychoanalysis/mental health community, we as a group bonded over our professional identity as psychologists dedicated to working with the military. This identity helped build strong connections within our group, mirroring the attachments our clients formed within their "brotherhood of arms."

The rapid, violent eruption of war following the Russian invasion in February 2022 did not catch any of us connected to this group by surprise. Thus, within the first week, we resumed the Intervision group, beginning to meet three times a week for a month and now continuing our ongoing Intervision groups weekly. We opened our group doors to all mental health and medical professionals who were involved in volunteering their support for the military defenders of Ukraine. Moreover, our Intervision group now found ourselves working not just with experienced and trained Ukrainian military service members but with numerous Ukrainians who were recently recruited and volunteer soldiers who, before the invasion, were IT specialists, engineers, restaurant chefs, teachers, and so forth. In this chapter, we further describe our Intervision group work, focusing on our setting, principals, and intricate psychological dynamics we observed in our meetings. In addition to expanding an understanding of the role and function of Intervision groups, we also hope to offer a glimpse into psychological work during the war.

Resilience amidst Chaos: Keeping Setting Alive in Times of War

During the first months after the invasion, when we met three times a week (Monday, Wednesday, and Friday evenings), the group primarily functioned as a support group for us as individuals, aiding us in navigating the overwhelming flow of emotions that accompanied such tumultuous times. In many ways, our experiences mirrored those of our patients' experiences during this crisis—the war brought us together, urging us to rekindle dormant connections and extend the invitation to predominantly virtual spaces for patients who also found themselves vulnerable. Each of our gatherings lasted one to two hours. However, as we gradually found means to cope, we realized it was important to shift the group setting and processes, prompting us to embrace change. In April of 2022, we started meeting weekly for an hour and a half to discuss emerging cases within the enlarged group (new members entered the group), into which new participants were welcomed. Because our meetings took place on Wednesday nights, many of us also felt connected to The Wednesday Psychological Society in Vienna at Freud's home, which was founded by Freud and a group of early psychoanalysts in 1902 but which actively functioned through the events of World War I. This group tradition, initiated in early psychoanalysis, inspired us, connecting us to an enduring practice that was larger than ourselves. We felt a vitality that transcends our immediate group dynamics and extends to our profound attachment to psychoanalysis as a practice.

Group Settings and Its Containing Function

Because of the conditions of war (e.g., safety) and interspersed locations of our participants who volunteer in hospitals, frontline areas, and other counseling centers, we remain meeting online. Each Intervision group begins with 10 minutes dedicated to warm welcoming, checking in about our well-being, and discussing any specific questions. Unlike other groups, which might skip such introductions, it enables participants to join the online group, engage in an introduction circle if new participants have entered, and overcome any internet connection issues frequently encountered in Ukraine nowadays (Figure 14.1). Once the initial 10 minutes have elapsed, we refrain from allowing additional participants to join in order not to compromise the integrity and trust within the group.

Remarkably, these initial 10 minutes serve as a space for a pre-case play, allowing the dynamic of upcoming cases to unfold. We deliberately refrain from scheduling case presentations in order to provide space for discussing urgent case material. Given that we are volunteers, we often find ourselves uncertain about when and from whom a request for psychological support may come; in our meetings, the case presentations are similarly unstructured. Typically, during the greeting phase, someone volunteers to present their case. Over the course of two years, there have been only two instances where

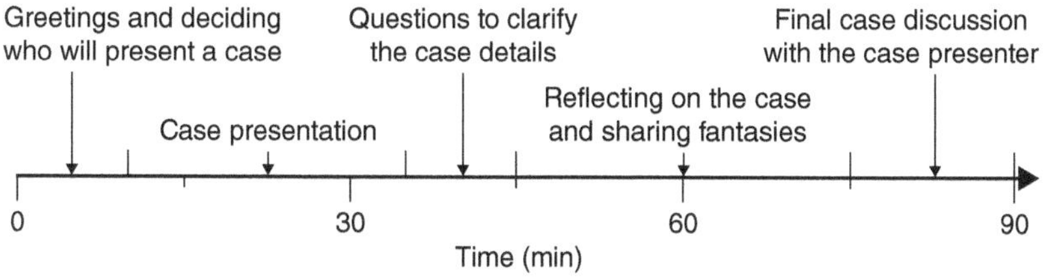

Figure 14.1 Schematic Outline of the Intervision Group Settings.

the group ended early due to the absence of a case. It is not uncommon for individuals to join without the intention of presenting a case, often prefacing their participation with a hesitant phrase such as, "Well, I don't have a case to present, I just want to ask…"—which often leads to fruitful case discussions.

As an example, recently, such a tentative question led to a profound group discussion about the ambiguous loss experienced by the wife of a Ukrainian serviceman. She is trapped in the tormenting uncertainty of whether her husband is dead or held captive by the Russians. Her life and the development of her three-year-old daughter were abruptly halted in March 2022 when her husband disappeared without a trace. Recognizing the child's plight, feeling neglected and deprived of attention by her distraught mother, the therapist felt compelled to intervene. Subsequently, the group identified a parallel between the pre-case group introduction comments (i.e., lack of clarity) and reflection of the mother's inability to function for herself and her child. Much like the therapist found the courage to "ask a simple question," the mother could only muster the strength to seek help for her daughter, remaining unapproachable herself when it came to her self-care and capacity to embrace life.

Typically in our groups, after the introduction, we proceed with the case presentation, which takes up to 20 minutes. We do not follow prescribed protocols for case presentations. Instead, we encourage a free narrative style, which has naturally evolved in our group. Typically, presenters now tend to follow a rough framework, commencing with a demographic background of the patient, followed by the circumstances that led to their engagement and the nature of their inquiry. They then outline the settings and number of sessions, providing available case descriptions. In the end, the therapist asks the group for specific help. Such help may be in sharing relevant experience or particular techniques; help may focus on aiding the practitioner to understand dynamics. Quite often, help is focused on normalizing the feelings of dealing with cases where specific rules or adages do not apply, which can make many of us practitioners of being "bad therapists".

Next, we continue with the questions aimed at clarifying case circumstances. These queries can encompass various aspects, including inquiries about the patient, the dynamics of the therapeutic process, or the therapist's emotions and countertransference. Duration of this group subsection can fluctuate from just a few minutes when there are no further questions, and the group eagerly transitions into a discussion to as long as 15 minutes when the group continues to pose questions seemingly insatiably, reluctant to move on to the case discussion. In the latest matter, the time restraints, as the reality principle, reminded the participants, and the group is encouraged to engage in dialogue rather than solely focusing on questions.

Discussions during our Intervision groups are held as having the utmost significance, taking up at least 30 minutes, during which each participant is encouraged to share their ideas, fantasies, associations, and so forth. All members must maintain a commitment to professionalism, care, and tactfulness when discussing the work of others because our primary objective is to provide support and guidance rather than exacerbate any challenges faced by the therapist. Our group comprises therapists from diverse backgrounds, ranging from individuals in formal psychoanalytic training to clinicians who practice positive psychology, Rogerian client-centered approach, and hypnotherapy, alongside individuals who have only studied psychology at an undergraduate level. This diversity of orientations enables us to examine cases from myriad perspectives, preventing us from being confined to a narrow understanding of each unique situation.

Notably, cases where patients employ projective identification as their primary defense mechanism frequently arise within our group. This phenomenon is particularly prevalent when working in a volunteer capacity with military personnel and individuals who have suffered war trauma. Projective identification seems to be the sole communicative tool for patients who are otherwise unable to express themselves in relation to their traumatic experience (Ogden, 2018). Furthermore, in projective identification, the aspect of self-projection onto the therapist and subsequently inflicting suffering upon them is often a suppressed aspect of the patient's psyche that requires attention for the individual to attain continued human existence.

Often, such patients only attend a few sessions because, for them, sessions are marked by compelled feelings to rid themselves of a nagging issue rising within themselves. Identifying projective identification can be challenging, even for seasoned professionals. I (Lukyanova) experienced this defense for the first time without understanding what it was or how to address it, leading to several days of internal turmoil as I grappled with the sensation of feeling like a sadist who needed to inflict physical suffering among the enemy. This process occurred while I was working with a Ukrainian soldier back in 2015. Having navigated such an unpleasant experience and knowing how to overcome it and where to seek help. I became committed to assisting other clinicians in avoiding falling into projective identification. Our group often serves as a support system in dealing with this phenomenon. Through a collaborative effort of sharing associations and fantasies and drawing upon our collective experience and knowledge, we can identify even the most complex cases and aid therapists in working through them.

In other instances, the group can present the therapist with entirely new insights about the case, revealing hidden material between the words and images. Sometimes, an excessive identification with the client impedes even the most experienced clinicians among us from objectively considering critical issues, such as the client's suicidal ideations. Alternatively, in specific cases, this identification causes therapists to become overly immersed in emotions, neglecting their professional knowledge. For instance, the group once reminded the therapist that victims of torture experience a breakdown of psychological and physical boundaries, which inevitably infiltrates therapeutic settings' breakdown, mirroring the patient's state of captivity. These examples offer just a glimpse into the extensive work undertaken by our groups, showcasing one of the generative aspects of our collaborative efforts.

The final part of the Intervision group entails continuing the discussion, now joined by the therapist initially presenting the case. At first, the therapist is invited to provide feedback to the group members and share the emotions accompanying each comment or select observations. This phase is dynamic, welcoming everyone to contribute ideas, yet under the guidance of the reality principle represented by the therapist, who has had direct contact with the real patient rather than merely a drawn representation. Typically, this segment concludes with warm farewells and promises to reconvene the following week.

Each segment of the Intervision group contributes to the unfolding case—beginning with the welcoming conversation during the initial 10 minutes and culminating in the closing discussion at the end of the 1.5-hour session. With each unique case, the patient's story gradually unfolds, starting from the moment the group convenes. Ultimately, the aim is to assist clinicians in comprehending the patient's situation, foster a sense of competence as therapists, and understand the reasons behind any fleeting moments of uncertainty that may arise during their practice.

Group Needs Both Parents

The majority of psychoanalytic groups operating during this War 2.0 (with 2014 as the first and 2022 as the second war wave) employ a dual-leadership structure. This approach, where therapists collaborate in pairs, much as a couple, when working with individuals who are severely traumatized, has been a feature of our Intervision group since its inception in 2014, when we first began assisting wounded military personnel. The dyadic relationship mirrors the dynamic of a parental couple caring for a child. This pattern emerges from the need of traumatized individuals to re-establish their sense of fundamental security and primary narcissism, often accompanied by mental regression in the presence of a parental couple. In times of war, the infringement upon Ukrainians' sense of basic security is pervasive, activating our attachment systems and heightening the imperative to support and restore everyone's sense of safety far beyond what is required under normal circumstances (Rudenko, 2023).

In our group, based on the findings from the experiences of some of our colleagues working with severely traumatized individuals, we observed that, at times, therapists find it exceedingly challenging to manage emotional and physiological countertransference on their own. When working with war victims, the profound horror and agony are frequently felt primarily at the bodily level. In these circumstances, the emotional aspect often remains elusive, and the therapist's body becomes actively involved, attempting to directly experience the patients' trauma without symbolizing it. There arises a necessity to communicate this transcendent, non-symbolic dissociated experience with another individual. In such instances, it would be beneficial to have a co-therapist who can serve as an observer and maintain the capacity for symbolic representation. This awareness is crucial because the therapist may unexpectedly identify with the patients when they attempt to focus on their own bodily experiences, as is typical in our psychotherapy practice with individuals who are less traumatized.

In a group, we also have two of us therapist leaders. In the group, all are encouraged not only to share their feelings, fantasies, and ideas with participants on an equal footing, but we, as facilitators, assume the roles of the parental figures. They cultivate a welcoming, supportive atmosphere, marking group milestones, encouraging active participation from others, and maintaining awareness of the time frame. Our Intervision group serves as a platform to collectively address and process the unspeakable or horrific experiences of the body and soul, providing containment and support.

Normalization of Feelings as the Main Goal

"All you need is love," sings John Lennon in the famous Beatles song. In the Ukrainian context today, we would argue that "All you need is to feel normal." Patients come to private and group therapy to feel normal. They want others to ensure that their feelings, reactions, thoughts, plans, or their absence are normal. Additionally, we, as a mental health specialist, are frontline workers for those who seek normality in a situation of war. People come to us and ask a direct question: "Is this normal?" And we are there to say yes. We respond over and over again: "This is a normal reaction to abnormal events. You are doing everything right. Follow your instincts." In our Intervision group, we repeat each other the same too, because we are all in the same space of normality-seeking.

We vividly remember the question of one of the therapists attending an Intervision group: "I could not hold myself back from crying when I identified with a wife of the military whose husband went missing. She was waiting for him, searching for videos on the internet that would confirm that he was still alive and that he was just waiting to be saved from captivity. I felt that there wasn't much hope left, but she was a living embodiment of Hope. I hugged her at the end of the session. I feel unprofessional for doing that." Just a few months later, this psychoanalyst, in fact, confirmed in the group that her patient's husband was indeed in captivity and had returned home. We are trained to be there for a patient but not to get involved. But the war put us, patients and therapists, in the same terrifying context. Is that normal?

Yet, was it normal when, in a post-war time of hunger in Vienna, patients were paying Freud with food? (Roazen, 2020). What of the time when Freud's patients knew that Marta Freud was sick and brought milk for her at a time when milk products were scarce? Did it jeopardize therapy to be more humane? (Roazen, 2020).

One of the unexpected aspects of working during the war was the normalization of not only feelings but also moral values and social positions held by the patients. One of our patients, a military wife, mentioned during a session the Facebook post I (Rudenko) published before our therapy meeting: "I am grateful to you for helping me and supporting me in my love for myself and in my relationship with my children. But it is much more important for me to see that you are a real person and that you boldly express your feelings in real life, not just in the office." This Facebook post was focused on support of the military and prisoners of war, attending rallies in their support. Only after such open posting on social media did the patient admit that she follows her therapist on social media.

In this case, the disclosure of the therapist's identity is, at times, treated as a violation of classical psychoanalysis. During the war, when the Russians have been constantly firing missiles and drones at us for over two years, death is everywhere, and fear and danger can unite or also divide people.

It is paramount for such times to discover people who share similar views, with whom you can easily identify and feel more secure in a community of people with the same values, even when such a person is also your therapist.

We are not suggesting here that we, as analysts, should cross all boundaries and become friends with our patients. As Nancy McWilliams (2023) reminded, one should first ask themselves if the action could be explained to the supervisor. Certainly, in typical circumstances, we must follow this therapeutic standard, but what of times of war? Psychoanalytic technical neutrality is also a consideration, commonly stressed, but what if therapists and patients share horrific realities and unsafe reactions? Nonetheless, we have found and affirmed in our group that we, as clinicians, had become far more present in the room with the patients because of the shared reality of war. Moreover, it is neither possible nor desirable to be removed and detached while calling it neutrality (Kernberg, 2016). We are trained not to take sides in the inner battles, but the sides in times of war in relation to the enemy must be taken clearly. Nonetheless, war brings changes that bring forth new ethical questions, and we need each other to discuss them.

We learned that the Intervision group is an ideal place to feel accepted. In the supervision group, multiple truths are held, which can be experienced by the Superego's tendency to hold on to a single truth. We all come together to present cases in a situation of equality. Certainly, in our group, some of us maintain group management or write chapters such as this. But we all mention how important it is to feel accepted and to have each other while holding different aspects of clinical reality.

We Are Standing under the Same Umbrella: Identity and Trauma

Before coalescing, every group, whether a small gathering or an entire societies, must establish a distinct identity. Identity is simultaneously the reason and the consequence of group functioning. When working with soldiers, psychologists strongly identify as "psychologists working with militaries," which automatically implies numerous ethical standards and underlying personal characteristics. Patients expect it from us as well.

A shared professional identity is an absolute prerequisite for a functional Intervision group, as it establishes a clear boundary for the trust-building process within the group. This identity is complex, as its nomenclature encompasses various underlying meanings, which we attempt to describe. Soldiers represent a specific group of people in every society, and their association forms a unique personal profile for individuals who choose to work with them.

Among those unique characteristics, which are mirroring our client's states and prerequisites, are:

> Patriotism and tolerance for the (necessary) splitting (between life and death, military and civil mental/physical life, enemy/own);
>
> High tolerance for war-related violence and/or personal posttraumatic growth experiences in the past;
>
> Constant contact with one's feelings, projections, and, crucially, countertransference;
>
> Knowledge of military slang and the specificity of military routines.

To serve one's country and to be ready willingly to sacrifice life, one must possess a profound patriotic sentiment. Ukrainians have borne witness to numerous courageous individuals who presented themselves at conscription centers, volunteering to join the military in the initial days of the invasion. Consequently, many of our patients and their loved ones were abruptly thrust into military service. This phenomenon is observable in private practices only during times of war. It was a harrowing yet captivating experience that unfolded in the early days of the conflict. This circumstance prompted numerous clinicians, who had never envisioned themselves in such a role or consciously chose not to work with the military, to find themselves addressing the needs of this particular group.

Many clinicians sought professional support and training to navigate the unfamiliar terrain. Much like our patients who were unexpectedly finding themselves among volunteers who are defending Ukraine, they were also searching for guidance and friendly advice for navigating the uncharted battlefields across the country. Indeed, numerous Ukrainian therapists and their clients found themselves in the same shoes, necessitating adjustments in size. Consequently, after February 24, 2022, many clients returned not to the comfortable couches but to the online meetings, adjusting to the new reality together with their psychologists. Just as in military service, where older colleagues provide training options for the younger generation, psychologists working with the military since 2014 have assisted less experienced colleagues. Our group emerged as one such space, extending a supportive environment for mutual growth and collaboration.

Another crucial aspect of successful work with military personnel is the specialist's ability to grapple with war-induced splitting. This includes clearly understanding who the aggressor and the victim are. Military individuals, equipped with mental fortitude and a solid comprehension of their boundaries, will likely discontinue working with a psychologist who attempts to instill doubts regarding the situation's right and wrong sides. Conversely, engaging with psychologists who maintain an undefined position can potentially be detrimental for military individuals who lack sufficient understanding of personal boundaries.

Tolerance to endure and absorb the continuum of emotions—pain, disgust, fear, excitement, and more—emanating from stories related to war-caused events and daily routines is crucial for psychologists working with the military. Frequently, in the early stages of establishing trust in the psychological partnership, military personnel will test a psychologist's ability to listen to their traumatic narratives, aiming to test their stress resilience. Once this trial is successfully passed, trust begins to take root.

Psychologists must perceive war as a duty essential for our physical and mental survival. Military individuals are inclined to confide in those who can bear the weight of the most horrifying and repugnant experiences they have endured. For a clinician, this necessitates a certain breadth of emotional resilience and life experience, underscoring the importance of personal therapy. Having a personal space where one can be authentic, vulnerable and contained is imperative—then constant, supportive therapy and supervision become essential. Just as our clients require our support, we, too, need someone to provide containment.

Furthermore, the process of working with trauma aims toward a specific goal—posttraumatic development, vividly mirrored in the metaphor of the Phoenix rising from the ashes. A soldier, stripped of the foundational sense of the value of human life, should rediscover this sentiment: a journey made possible through therapy guided by a therapist who has undergone such an experience. Similar to how children instinctively trust their parents in the process of upbringing, soldiers should develop trust in their therapist to accompany them on the path to healing and reflection on their trauma.

A clinician acquires this experiential understanding through their own therapeutic processes, facing profound losses, sometimes as fundamental as those endured by our patients. In this context, Intervision groups emerge as an ideal space for acceptance, serving as a container for the emotional challenges encountered in this line of work. When working with soldiers, the clinician often functions as a fragmented part of the psyche, tasked with the role of feeling function. Soldiers, by the nature of their duty, are often constrained from expressing their emotions; they must focus on the act of fighting. Consequently, we consciously refrain from provoking emotional work but engage with their feelings unconsciously. In a sense, we act as radar, capturing a spectrum of our client's emotions and sorting through them to discern the genuine from the noise.

Case Presentation

Here, we would like to provide an example of a military patient who suppressed his feelings, while the therapist would experience and process those abandoned emotions.

The patient endured the loss of many comrades throughout the decade-long conflict between Russia and Ukraine. He sustained injuries but bravely returned to the battlefield. Concurrently, his mother battled a prolonged illness at home. Six months following her passing, he found himself unable to manage his growing irritation and anger towards those around him. Such emotions and behavior were uncharacteristic of him, leading to his admission to a psychiatric facility. With the aid of medication, he experienced improvement, and his outbursts of unprovoked aggression towards fellow soldiers ceased. However, along with the aggression, his zest for life diminished. He no longer found joy in anything, lacked desire, and became indifferent to the prospect of his own mortality.

During our sessions, I (Rudenko) grappled with an overwhelming sense of longing and sorrow. Often, after the patient departed, I found solace in releasing pent-up tears, overcome by profound sadness. Yet, the patient remained unaffected by grief or melancholy, instead expressing only emptiness and detachment. He confided in feeling immense guilt and shame regarding the multitude of deaths he had witnessed but never grief. Similarly, he struggled to mourn the loss of his mother, as the capacity for grieving had yet to materialize.

I presented this case at the Intervision group meeting. As the group delved into this case, each participant experienced a range of emotions, including sadness and grief, which found a place within our discussions. In instances involving military personnel, the conventional process of grieving for the loss of loved ones is disrupted. The overwhelming nature of such loss often fragments, rendering it inaccessible to the conscious psyche. Instead, feelings of guilt, shame, and profound rage tend to emerge as they are perceived as more manageable or socially acceptable.

It was only through the group dynamic that I found the opportunity to acknowledge, identify, and integrate the myriad emotions associated with loss. Subsequently, in the following session with this patient, we enabled him to commence the grieving process for his mother. Furthermore, as he shared his experiences of losing comrades, he transitioned from self-punitive guilt to experiencing the profound sadness and grief inherent in these irreparable losses. Gradually, he reclaimed his customary vitality and zest for life.

In the example above, projection and countertransference were used extensively. When comprehended and reflected upon, these psychological mechanisms aid our clients in healing. To effectively navigate this terrain, the specialist necessitates specific experience, supervision, and the supportive camaraderie of colleagues in the field, as achieved in an Intervision group.

An intriguing observation within our group's work is the prevalence of cases where specialists contend with projective identification. This significant phenomenon serves as a remarkably successful avenue for our patients to convey their emotions and the intricate state of the psyche when words alone prove inadequate. Indeed, what aids in earning the trust and respect of soldiers lies within the realm of language. Much like the importance for us specialists to communicate effectively through professional jargon, it holds equal significance for military personnel to sense that they can place their trust in us. This connection is encapsulated in their everyday slang, where the subtle nuances of their daily routine are embedded. When we comprehend this language and refrain from interrupting our clients for every unfamiliar term, the stories we hear can be fully and unadulteratedly expressed.

Conclusion

Intervision groups serve as invaluable tools for specialists to convene and reflect on cases and the emotions they evoke, especially during times of war, when mental health professionals confront an immense amount of ambiguity and challenges stemming not only from the inner world of the patient but also from external, uncontrollable events. Intervision groups provide new clinicians with a foundation and support from more experienced colleagues.

Established in 2014 and reinstated in February 2022, our Intervision group brings together specialists from diverse backgrounds, operating within a psychoanalytic framework. Its promising dynamic hinges on the shared identity of working with soldiers, fostering knowledge-sharing and mutual support as we await victory.

We conclude with a message of hope, encapsulated in a dream one of us (Rudenko) had on the night War 2.0 began:

> I found myself sunbathing at the seaside with my two children and husband. The sun shined brightly overhead as I held my smartphone in hand. Suddenly, a colossal wave emerged from the sea, towering like a wall. Despite my fear, I clutched my younger child's hand tightly as the wave engulfed us. After a while, we were washed ashore. Though my husband and daughter were not by my side, I felt reassured knowing they were safe and that we would reunite soon. Despite the ordeal, the sun's brightness remained unchanged, instilling a sense of calm within me. I firmly believe that, in time, all will be well.

References

Kernberg, O. F. (2016). The four basic components of psychoanalytic technique and derived psychoanalytic psychotherapies. *World Psychiatry*, 15(3), 287–288. https://doi.org/10.1002/wps.20368

McWilliams, N. (2023). For my Ukrainian colleagues on a painful anniversary: Some heartfelt ideas for maintaining practice under fire. *Ukrainian Psychoanalytic Journal*, 1(1), 7–13. https://doi.org/10.32782/upj/2023-1-2

Ogden, T. H. (2018). *Projective identification and psychotherapeutic technique*. In Routledge eBooks. https://doi.org/10.4324/9780429478574

Pustovoyt, M. (2023). Interpreting crisis while in crisis (reflections on psychoanalytic work in hybrid warfare). *Ukrainian Psychoanalytic Journal*, 1(1), 21–26. https://doi.org/10.32782/upj/2023-1-4

Roazen, P. (2020). *Brother animal: The story of Freud and Tausk*. Routledge.

Rudenko, R. (2023). Traveling through the worlds: New challenges in therapy with children, adolescents, and their families during the war. *Psychoanalytic Psychology*, 40(4), 243–246. https://doi.org/10.1037/pap0000481

Staempfli, A., & Fairtlough, A. (2019). Intervision and professional development: An exploration of a peer-group reflection method in social work education. *The British Journal of Social Work*, 49(5), 1254–1273.

Chapter 15

International and National Psychoanalytic Initiatives in Wartime Ukraine

History of 2022–2023

Alexander A. Lupis, Marianna Tkalych, and Mariana Velykodna

In response to the 2022 Russian invasion of Ukraine, local and foreign psychoanalytic societies and groups launched various initiatives to address the issues related both to wartime and previous post-Soviet or post-imperial legacies. This chapter introduces the history of these initiatives of 2022–2023 through four main topics: (1) addressing the mental health crisis; (2) supporting the ongoing psychoanalytic practice in wartime; (3) promoting the voice of Ukrainian psychodynamic clinicians and scholars for the international audience; and (4) building the sustainable development of psychoanalysis in Ukraine. As the authors of this chapter are psychodynamic scholars affiliated with the National Psychological Association of Ukraine (NPA), the main focus will be given to the initiatives associated with NPA, with an attempt to cover some other significant processes launched by other professional societies and institutions.

Addressing the Mental Health Crisis

The need for mental health assistance within the population increased dramatically following the large-scale invasion of Ukraine in February 2022 (Lushchak et al., 2023), often compounding the mental health issues that had developed in response to the initial 2014 Russian invasion of eastern Ukraine (Tkalych et al., 2023). The mental health system in Ukraine, which existed until that moment, however, could not provide the required amount and quality of care to a broader segment of the population (Seleznova et al., 2023). Several non-governmental organizations established in 2014 working with war victims, active-duty soldiers, and veterans continued and intensified their activities but also could not cover the rapidly growing needs for

DOI: 10.4324/9781032660257-16

care (e.g., Fedorets, 2023). The intensification of the war led many patients (clients) and mental health clinicians to lose their homes, jobs, and financial security. While some analysts reported they were able to continue working partly free of charge (Rudenko, 2023; Velykodna et al., 2023), others lost almost all their patients and were seeking jobs and advanced training to provide crisis counseling and other trauma-oriented psychological interventions (Palii et al., 2023). The Ukrainian psychoanalytic community expressed an interest in expanding clinical training and providing as much help as possible to the population affected by war (Velykodna et al., 2022).

In the spring of 2022, NPA leaders sought to address the gap between the growing demand and limited availability of mental healthcare services by securing international funding – from the United Nations Development Programme, the European Union, and the governments of Denmark and Canada) to launch a psychological hotline in Ukraine and 21 neighboring countries (Palii et al., 2023). Five psychodynamic practitioners who are members of NPA's Psychoanalytic Psychology and Psychotherapy Division of NPA joined the hotline and have worked there throughout the war – one as a coordinator (Tetiana Dzisiak) and four psychological assistance providers (Sergii Ugrium, Olga Karpenko, Olga Balmen, Kateryna Edelieva).

In parallel, two members of NPA's Psychoanalytic Psychology and Psychotherapy Division (Volodymyr Mamko and Valeriy Dorozhkin) organized their independent mental health projects in partnership with the Division and involved more psychodynamic specialists in them. In March 2022, Volodymyr Mamko launched the Professional Supervision Institute in Kyiv, where psychoanalysts worked both online and locally in person with war-exposed and injured civilians and soldiers. The clinicians were provided with daily support groups and supervision sessions, which also included training on crisis interventions and trauma care (Yevlanova, 2023). Valeriy Dorozhkin's "Psychologists at war" project organized a team of mental health professionals, including psychodynamic ones, worked directly in the recently liberated territories that have been occupied by Russian troops since August 2022. This project provided medical and psychosocial aid in villages and small towns as well as supervision sessions for clinicians.

During the spring and fall of 2022, NPA rapidly expanded online training initiatives for NPA members throughout Ukraine, and especially to support counselors working for NPA's national and international crisis hotline. These included courses taught by Dr. Marcio Pereira on behalf of the Order of Portuguese Psychologists (Ordem dos Psicólogos Portugueses), Professor

Jane L. Ireland and Kimberley McNeill of the University of Lancashire, Dr. Iva Bicanic of the University Medical Centre Utrecht, Thomas Ch. Weber and his colleagues from the Vienna-based Institute of Neuropsychotherapy, Dr. Shanna Williams of McGill University, Emeritus of Clinical Psychology Western Carolina University Prof. David McCord, as well as participation in the Global Summit Collective Trauma 2022.

Some of NPA's partners prepared extensive training for clinicians in Ukraine. Dr. Marc Hillbrand of the Yale University School of Medicine and colleagues from Section XII – Clinical Emergencies and Crises of APA Division 12 – Society of Clinical Psychology, organized crisis counseling seminars. Dr. Stephen Cozza of the US Department of Defense's medical school in Bethesda, Maryland, the Uniformed Services University of the Health Sciences (USUHS), organized what is an ongoing series of training courses on supporting children from military families. And the Society for Psychotherapy Research prepared an entire conference for Ukrainian clinicians on self-care.

Support of Psychoanalytic Practice in Ukraine

In addition to the abovementioned efforts to provide Ukrainian clinicians with appropriate crisis interventions and to train psychodynamic practitioners with relevant non-analytic clinical skills, some initiatives specifically focused on supporting psychoanalytic practice in wartime. These were support groups, continuous education pieces and supervision projects.

On the second day of the large-scale invasion, February 25, 2022, NPA's Psychoanalytic Psychology and Psychotherapy Division launched its first online support group that was led by Valeriy Dorozhkin, Olga Pavlovska, Natalia Turbina, and Natalia Nalyvaiko. This 2-hour group met weekly with two rotating group co-leaders during the first three months. Later the group changed its frequency to every fortnight during summer and met monthly in fall of 2022 until the massive blackouts throughout Ukraine and then stopped. The group had an open call for participants among Ukrainian psychoanalytic practitioners and candidates and provided a safe space for containing their thoughts, feelings, worries, and inquiries.

During the same period, support groups and large analytic groups were launched by other psychoanalytic societies within Ukraine. For instance, the International Virtual Large Group began their work to support Ukrainian psychotherapists, which was offered by the Tel Aviv Institute of Modern

Psychoanalysis, the Greek Institute of Relational and Group Psychotherapy, in cooperation with the Kyiv International School of Relational Psychoanalysis and Psychotherapy. There were also large and small groups that met every week, fortnight, or month, launched by the Ukrainian Union of Psychotherapists and the Association of Psychotherapists and Psychoanalysts of Ukraine. The Melanie Klein Trust in collaboration with the Ukrainian Psychoanalytic Society, also launched a support group called Help for Helpers.

Within the support group provided by the NPA's Psychoanalytic Psychology and Psychotherapy Division till fall 2022, it became evident that the request for support has changed and was more appropriate for supervision. NPA Psychoanalytic Psychology and Psychotherapy Division members who were not attending this group were also expressing that they would benefit of having a supervision group or even groups. The problem was that the extremely high demand for help from people resulted in certified specialists and supervisors being overloaded with clinical work and being less available to support their colleagues at precisely the time when candidates and early career professionals desperately needed supervision for their crisis-related work. Furthermore, psychoanalysis and psychoanalytic psychotherapy training programs often were halted for at least six months (Velykodna et al., 2023). Because of the high need in therapy within the population, candidates were forced to start practicing before completing their training and certification and also needed supervision, including for resolving ethical dilemmas (Velykodna et al., 2023). Thus, there was a significant increase in the demand for psychotherapy in Ukraine, as well as a corresponding increase in demand for continuing education and supervision among therapists.

The continuous education in the psychoanalytic approach during the war has varied in forms from lectures and seminars to brief courses, reading groups, and practically oriented conferences. Educational lectures conducted by distinguished psychoanalytic therapists provided Ukrainian analysts not only with useful theory but also with an important feeling of connectedness and solidarity with the broader professional world. For instance, Dr. Nancy McWilliams held a special lecture for Ukrainian colleagues in February of 2023 in support of specialists in Ukraine working with the psychological consequences of the Russian invasion. In May 2023 Dr. Katie Lewis, director of research at the Austen Riggs Center in Stockbridge, Massachusetts, conducted a training on psychoanalytic approaches to suicide and suicide intervention. In fall 2023, Dr. Salman Akhtar provided the audience of the NPA members with a lecture on the role of silence in the psychoanalytic process.

An important issue was the significant need for couples and family therapy since the war started, as many husbands and fathers were fighting in the military while mothers and children stayed home and men were not allowed to leave the country while many mothers and children fled to safer places either in Western Ukraine or Central Europe. NPA's Psychoanalytic Psychology and Psychotherapy Division addressed this gap by partnering with the Washington Baltimore Center for Psychoanalysis in the summer of 2023 so that Noa Ashman and Dr. Carolyn Ratner-Fitzgerald could teach an online class in psychoanalytic couples therapy for 40 Ukrainian psychodynamic practitioners. Moreover, the Washington-Baltimore Center for Psychoanalysis invited the division members to participate freely in all their educational activities for the current academic year, like seminars and colloquiums.

The Psychoanalytic Psychology and Psychotherapy Division of the NPA also held clinical seminars on working with non-neurotic issues (Olga Pavlovska, Natalia Turbina, Nina Kokoilo, Sergii Ugrium) and on psychoanalytic investigations of speech and language in relation to unspeakable (Olena Medvedieva, Yehor Butsykin, Elina Yevlanova, Natalia Nalyvaiko, Mariana Velykodna) and launched continuous reading groups focused on Ukrainian translations of Freud's (led by Yehor Butsykin and Elina Yevlanova) and Lacan's texts (led by Olena Medvedieva). We also organized three conferences that addressed the issues raised from practicing in wartime: "Psychoanalysis Revised by War. Ethics, Clinics, and Personal Experience" (October 2022), "Ethical Challenges in Psychoanalytic Practice in Wartime" (April 2023), and "Psychoanalysis on Time" (November 2023). No less important is that our monthly online lectorium, "Psychoanalysis. Open Space," led by Yulia Vizniuk, continued throughout the war after a short pause.

Most other psychoanalytic societies in Ukraine also opened their training for other colleagues. The Ukrainian Psychoanalytic Society (IPA study group) during 2022–2023 held six international meetings, which combined both educational and supportive purposes as included oral presentations and discussions. The Association of Interdisciplinary Childhood Support PARTUS (Ukraine), in partnership with the association La Cause des bébés (France), has started open seminars for psychoanalysts, psychologists, doctors, and nurses aimed at working with children and their parents from Ukraine who are experiencing trauma, using a psychoanalytic lens on the issues of separation, parting, abandonment, infants' and toddlers' symptoms. The Association of Psychotherapists and Psychoanalysts of Ukraine, in cooperation with the Psychoanalytic Assistance in Crisis and Emergency Situations Committee of the International Psychoanalytic Association

(PACE IPA), held a series of seminars "Trauma and Childhood" provided by specialists with many years of clinical experience working with children and adolescents who have suffered severe psychological trauma.

Many international societies invited Ukrainian colleagues to attend their online conferences free of charge. For instance, in June 2022 the Irene Society in the Czech Republic invited Ukrainians to "Prague Talking 2022: Apocalypse and the Survival of Hope." In May 2023, Ukrainian psychodynamic clinicians were invited to the conference entitled "Reciprocal Resilience: Working with Children, Adolescents and Their Parents" held by the Institute of Counselling and Psychoanalytic Studies in New Jersey, USA.

The increased need for psychoanalytic supervision led Dr. Alexander Lupis to reach out to Dr. Sara Hedlund, a professor of psychology and supervision trainer at George Washington University in Washington, DC. Dr. Hedlund and NPA colleagues established a supervision process group with 20 members of the Psychoanalytic Psychology and Psychotherapy Division in December 2022 that met to discuss challenges in providing psychoanalytic interventions during the war. This group still works in 2024. In the winter of 2022–2023, Dr. Lupis also reached out to a team of psychoanalytic supervisors affiliated with Boston-based psychoanalyst Dr. Cris Ratiner and her nonprofit Eyra Psychosocial Assistance. Dr. Ratiner supported a project launched by Volodymyr Mamko that paired Ukrainian clinicians with US-based psychoanalytic supervisors. Noa Ashman and Dr. Carolyn Ratner-Fitzgerald from the Washington Baltimore Center for Psychoanalysis have also provided 10 Ukrainian couple therapists from NPA's Psychoanalytic Psychology and Psychotherapy Division with an ongoing supervision group.

Voice of Ukrainian Psychodynamic Clinicians and Scholars for the International Audience

Many colleagues abroad were eager to better understand the 2022 Russian invasion of Ukraine that had shocked and surprised the world. Unfortunately, this created favorable conditions for the spread of Russian propaganda (Romanov, 2023), which denied many of the brutal realities of the invasion (Romanov, 2024). It was, therefore, very important for Ukrainian experts to provide their own perspectives for foreign audiences. Such speeches and texts not only highlighted current events and their historical significance but also informed colleagues about what help can be provided to Ukraine and psychoanalytic practitioners here.

Already in April 2022, the editors of the journal *Psychodynamic Practice* invited the authors from the Psychoanalytic Psychology and Psychotherapy Division of the NPA to add a brief concluding commentary about facing war to the conference report submitted for publication before the full-scale invasion (Velykodna et al., 2022). In June 2022, a discussion "Psychoanalysis under conditions of war" was organized by the Freud Foundation US and the Sigmund Freud Museum, Vienna, encompassing an international group of speakers: F. Davoine (France); O. Filts (Ukraine); G. Fromm (the USA); and J. Wolff Bernstein as a moderator.

In July 2022, the *International Journal of Psychoanalysis* published a Letter from the Ukrainian Psychoanalytic Society (Mirza & Romanov, 2022). Dr. Alexander Lupis authored an article in March 2023 describing NPA's training programs and leadership for Harvard University's Ukrainian Research Institute. That same month, he co-authored an article with NPA president Dr. Valeriia Palii in the Psychiatric Times about the need for mental health care reforms and funding to be prioritized in post-war reconstruction.

In April 2023, seven members of the Psychoanalytic Psychology and Psychotherapy Division of the NPA – Mariana Velykodna, Natalia Nalyvaiko, Valeriy Dorozhkin, Elina Yevlanova, Olga Pavlovska, Ruslana Rudenko, and Yehor Butsykin – were invited by the Washington Baltimore Center for Psychoanalysis to speak at the special event accredited by the American Psychoanalytic Association on "Rethinking Psychoanalytic Practice in wartime." This event aroused the great interest of attendees. The presentations made a big impression, so speakers were invited to publish them as papers in a special section of the journal *Psychoanalytic Psychology* with an introduction of Kevin Meehan and Oksana Yakushko and a closing commentary by Nancy McWilliams in fall 2023. In December 2023, the project *Psychoanalytic Authors on the Couch* published a video conversation between Oksana Yakushko and Mariana Velykodna regarding this special section (Yakushko & Velykodna, 2023).

The International Forum of Psychoanalytic Education in the USA invited Ukrainian colleagues from the Psychoanalytic Psychology and Psychotherapy Division of the NPA to speak at two panel discussions with a general title, "Psychoanalytic practice in times of war," in May and July of 2023. Ukrainian psychoanalytic specialists – Olga Pavlovska, Valeriy Dorozhkin, Volodymyr Mamko, Elina Yevlanova, Natalia Nalivayko, Ruslana Rudenko, and Sergii Ugrium – presented their experience as speakers and Mariana Velykodna and Oksana Yakushko (a psychologist and psychoanalyst originally from Ukraine who has lived and worked in the USA for many years in Santa Barbara, CA) were moderators of this event.

To support more voices from Ukraine to be heard, in the spring of 2023, Oksana Yakushko, together with Ukraine-based psychoanalyst Mariana Velykodna, conducted a series of four webinars designed specifically for the NPA members. Seminars were devoted to the preparation of research papers and book proposals in psychology for publication in English, as well as work with editors and book publishers.

In June 2023, the Department of Psychology at Long Island University in Brooklyn, New York, together with the NPA, launched a joint research colloquium where scholars from Ukraine, including psychoanalytically oriented ones, presented their current understandings of the different kinds of psychological impact of war on the citizens in and refugees from Ukraine. In the same month, due to the efforts of Darren Haber (USA), *Psychoanalysis, Self and Context* journal published a special issue, "Ukrainian Voices in Wartime," with contributions from psychoanalytic therapists from the Ukrainian Union of Psychotherapists and the Ukrainian Confederation of Psychoanalytic Psychotherapies along with the commentaries of foreign colleagues (e.g., Kechur & Haber, 2023).

In July 2023, after the consideration of their submitted book proposal, members of the Psychoanalytic Psychology and Psychotherapy Division of the NPA received an official offer to publish a book on psychoanalytic practice during the war from Routledge. Mariana Velykodna, Oksana Yakushko, and Adrienne Harris were assigned as the editors of this book. We considered this proposal as an opportunity to contribute to the psychoanalytic understanding of mental processes during crisis events, share practical findings of Ukrainian psychoanalytic psychotherapists, introduce the reader to Ukrainian specialists in the field of psychoanalysis, psychoanalytic psychotherapy and psychology, and inform the public more about the war in Ukraine. However, we did not stop at this point and made several other publications regarding the practice in wartime (e.g., Velykodna et al., 2023; Velykodna et al., 2024).

Finally, in the fall of 2023, the *Psychoanalytic Inquiry* journal accepted the proposal for a special issue devoted to Russia's war against Ukraine based on the contributions of Ukrainian psychoanalytic scholars who represent different psychoanalytic societies – Mariana Velykodna, Mykhaylo Pustovoyt, Oleksandr Fedorets, Petro Harmish, Vladimir Lagutin, Valeriy Dorozhkin – together with Sergio Benvenuto and Oksana Yakushko. These papers are currently in press.

Building the Sustainable Development of Psychoanalysis in Ukraine

The processes described above are more about responding to the war and engaging the international audience in understanding and countering it. But it was also important to invest in the broader development of psychoanalysis in Ukraine, especially through its inclusion into a global psychoanalytic community to separate more effectively from the Soviet and post-Soviet past much affected by Russian imperial culture and ideology (Butsykin, 2023). Apart from the issues of psychoanalytic training, which goes well within various Ukrainian professional associations affiliated with distinguished international societies, three processes could facilitate this transition: (1) increasing the visibility and credibility of Ukrainian psychoanalysts and the promotion of their texts written in the Ukrainian language; (2) providing Ukrainian analysts with increased access to the texts of psychoanalysts worldwide in English or in Ukrainian translation; (3) promoting psychoanalysis to be recognized as evidence-based practice within Ukraine; and (4) supporting international scholarships, fellowships, and other exchange.

Foremost, during the war many representatives of various Ukrainian psychoanalytic communities began to speak publicly more to international as well as to Ukrainian audiences, particularly in the media, as well as to give lectures and seminars to colleagues and to the general population. This showed that there are many psychoanalytic ideas that are worthy of attention and publication in the form of articles. Second, many scholars intensified their efforts to translate psychoanalytic books from English or other European languages. However, book translation and publication is a long and complicated process, while sometimes, having a translated paper is more of a priority.

Following this impression, in 2023, the members of the Psychoanalytic Psychology and Psychotherapy Division of the NPA launched the *Ukrainian Psychoanalytic Journal* – a peer-reviewed electronic open-access scholarly periodical recognized by Ukraine's Ministry of the Education and Science (Velykodna et al., 2024). Currently, the journal is supported by various psychoanalytic institutions and scholars and publishes original papers, commentaries, reviews, and translations in the Ukrainian language. No less important is that the journal contributes to the recognition of psychoanalytic practice as evidence-based. Due to the efforts of its authors and editorial board members, by the end of 2023, psychoanalytic therapy for the first time was added to an official list of methods with proven efficacy established by Ukraine's Ministry of Healthcare.

Since 2022, we sought ways for scholarships and fellowship programs for Ukrainian psychoanalytic therapists, both residential – for those who had to flee the country – and non-residential. In November 2022, Dr. Alexander Lupis reached out to the Committee on International Relations at the APA Division 39 – Society of Psychoanalysis and Psychoanalytic Psychology. They developed a plan to publicize the division's annual residential scholars program among colleagues in Ukraine, and several were accepted in the spring of 2023. Many clinicians were, however, unable to apply as they were not able to meet the requirement to attend the division's annual spring conference in the USA. As a result of this, the committee responded by creating a new temporary non-residential scholars program in the spring of 2023 for clinicians who were unable to travel, and the first group was accepted in the fall of 2023. The non-residential scholars' program became a permanent program in order to accommodate clinicians from Ukraine and from Gaza.

In 2023, 6 members of the Division passed the competitive selection of projects for the International Scholar Program of the Society for Psychoanalysis and Psychoanalytic Psychology (Division 39) of the American Psychological Association in 2023–2024. They are Anastasia Tokareva, Mariana Velykodna, Oksana Arshevska-Guérin, Sergii Ugrium, Zoia Miroshnyk, and Yelyzaveta Davoian. This fellowship provides opportunities for Ukrainian psychotherapists to have international membership in this division, access to the Psychoanalytic Electronic Publishing (PEP)-web psychoanalytic library, access to the division's publications, and personal mentoring support with monthly online meetings throughout the year to work on the project. In addition to the PEP-web library, we are grateful to the American Psychological Association for providing free access to the scientific database PsycINFO for NPA's members, which allowed Ukraine-based scholars and practitioners affected by war to seek relevant literature and distract from unbearable reality for reading.

Conclusions

At a time when Ukraine is facing an existential military invasion as well as daily missile attacks against cities far from the front lines, the initiatives described above have created, over the past two years, a new network of ongoing communication, connection, learning, and support between

Ukrainian and Western clinicians, as well as increased cooperation and support between Ukrainian clinicians. This intellectual and psychological network has both supported and learned from brave Ukrainian clinicians who are living through as well as simultaneously trying to heal the horrors of a brutal, genocidal war. Western clinicians have seen what may be in store for their own societies or for their own military forces if international support for Ukraine is limited and Russian military forces prevail and move onward toward the Baltics, Scandinavia, or Central Europe. Most importantly, this ongoing exchange of experiences and ideas among professional colleagues has improved the quality of mental healthcare care afforded to Ukrainian civilians and soldiers as the Ukrainian state and society struggle toward liberating their territory, pursuing criminal justice for perpetrators, and moving ahead with European integration.

As concluding remarks, we wish to express our gratitude to Ukrainian psychoanalytic specialists who maintain investing in Ukraine and its psychoanalytic present and future (e.g., Romanov, 2024), as well as to our foreign friends who support us in these unprecedented times.

References

Butsykin, Y. (2023). Translating psychoanalytic texts into Ukrainian: Discoveries and further steps. *Psychoanalytic Psychology*, 40(4), 261–265. https://doi.org/10.1037/pap0000483

Fedorets, O. (2023). Counseling on the front line: Insights from a Ukrainian doctor. *Psychoanalysis, Self and Context*, 18(3), 345–351. https://doi.org/10.1080/24720038.2023.2209129

Kechur, R., & Haber, D. (2023). An exchange with Roman Kechur: Preserving thinking during wartime. *Psychoanalysis, Self and Context*, 18(3), 364–378. https://doi.org/10.1080/24720038.2023.2203028

Lushchak, O., Velykodna, M., Bolman, S., Strilbytska, O., Berezovskyi, V., & Storey, K.B. (2023). Prevalence of stress, anxiety, and symptoms of post-traumatic stress disorder among Ukrainians after the first year of Russia invasion: A nationwide cross-sectional study. *The Lancet Regional Health – Europe*, 36, https://doi.org/10.1016/j.lanepe.2023.100773

Mirza, O., & Romanov, I. (2022). Letter from the Ukrainian psychoanalytic society. *The International Journal of Psychoanalysis*, 103(3), 427–430. https://doi.org/10.1080/00207578.2022.2066275

Palii, V., Velykodna, M., Pereira, M., McElvaney, R., Bernard, S., Klymchuk, V., Burlachuk, O., Lupis, A. A., Diatel, N., Ireland, J. L.; McNeill, K., Scarlet, J. L., Jaramillo-Sierra, A. L., Khoury, B., Sánchez Munar, D. R., Hedlund, S., Flanagan, T., LeBlanc, J., Agudelo Velez, D. M., & Gómez-Maquet, Y. (2023).

The experience of launching a psychological hotline across 21 countries to support Ukrainians in wartime. *Mental Health and Social Inclusion*. https://doi.org/10.1108/MHSI-04-2023-0040

Romanov, I. (2023). Contemporary propaganda and propagandistic states of mind: A psychoanalytic view. *Ukrainian Psychoanalytic Journal*, 1(3), 24–29. https://doi.org/10.32782/upj/2023-3-4

Romanov, I. (2024). Geschichte eines ukrainischen Psychoanalytikers. *Psyche*, 78(6), 508–534. https://doi.org/10.21706/ps-78-6-508

Rudenko, R. (2023). Traveling through the worlds: New challenges in therapy with children, adolescents and their families during the war. *Psychoanalytic Psychology*, 40(4). https://doi.org/10.1037/pap0000481

Seleznova, V., Pinchuk, I., Feldman, I., Virchenko, V., Wang, B. & Skokauskas, N. (2023). The battle for mental well-being in Ukraine: Mental health crisis and economic aspects of mental health services in wartime. *International Journal of Mental Health Systems*, 17(1), 28. https://doi.org/10.1186/s13033-023-00598-3

Tkalych, M., Snyadanko, I., Shapovalova, T., Falova, O., & Sokolova, I. (2023). Psychological rehabilitation of combatants in Ukraine from 2014 to 2021: Statistics and current status. *Acta Neuropsychologica*, 21(4), 441–455. https://doi.org/10.5604/01.3001.0054.0125

Velykodna, M., Butsykin, Y., Dorozhkin, V., Lupis, A., Melnychuk, T., Nalyvaiko, N., Pavlovska, O., Pustovoyt, M., Tkalych, M., & Yakushko, O. (2024). Inscribing a new page in the history of Ukrainian psychoanalysis during the wartime: The call for contributions. *International Journal of Applied Psychoanalytic Studies*. https://doi.org/10.1002/aps.1861

Velykodna, M., Dorozhkin, V., Nalyvaiko, N., Yevlanova, E. & Lunov, V. (2022) Life and death of psychoanalytic societies – Lessons from history and new prospects for unions: Conference report, Kyiv, Ukraine, 2021, *Psychodynamic Practice*, (3). https://doi.org/10.1080/14753634.2022.2064351

Velykodna, M., Nalyvaiko, N., Pavlovska, O., Arshevska-Guérin, O. & Butsykin, Y. (2023). Ethical challenges in psychoanalytic practice in wartime: Conference report, Kyiv, Ukraine, 2023. *Psychodynamic Practice*. https://doi.org/10.1080/14753634.2023.2258036

Yakushko, O. & Velykodna, M. (2023). Psychoanalysis and war: On witnessing Ukrainian psychoanalysts. *Psychoanalytic Authors on the Couch*. Episode 6. https://www.youtube.com/watch?v=uJ3fALxYV3M

Yevlanova, E. (2023). Professional supervision as therapists' self-care during wartime. *Psychoanalytic Psychology*, 30(4). https://doi.org/10.1037/pap0000486

Index

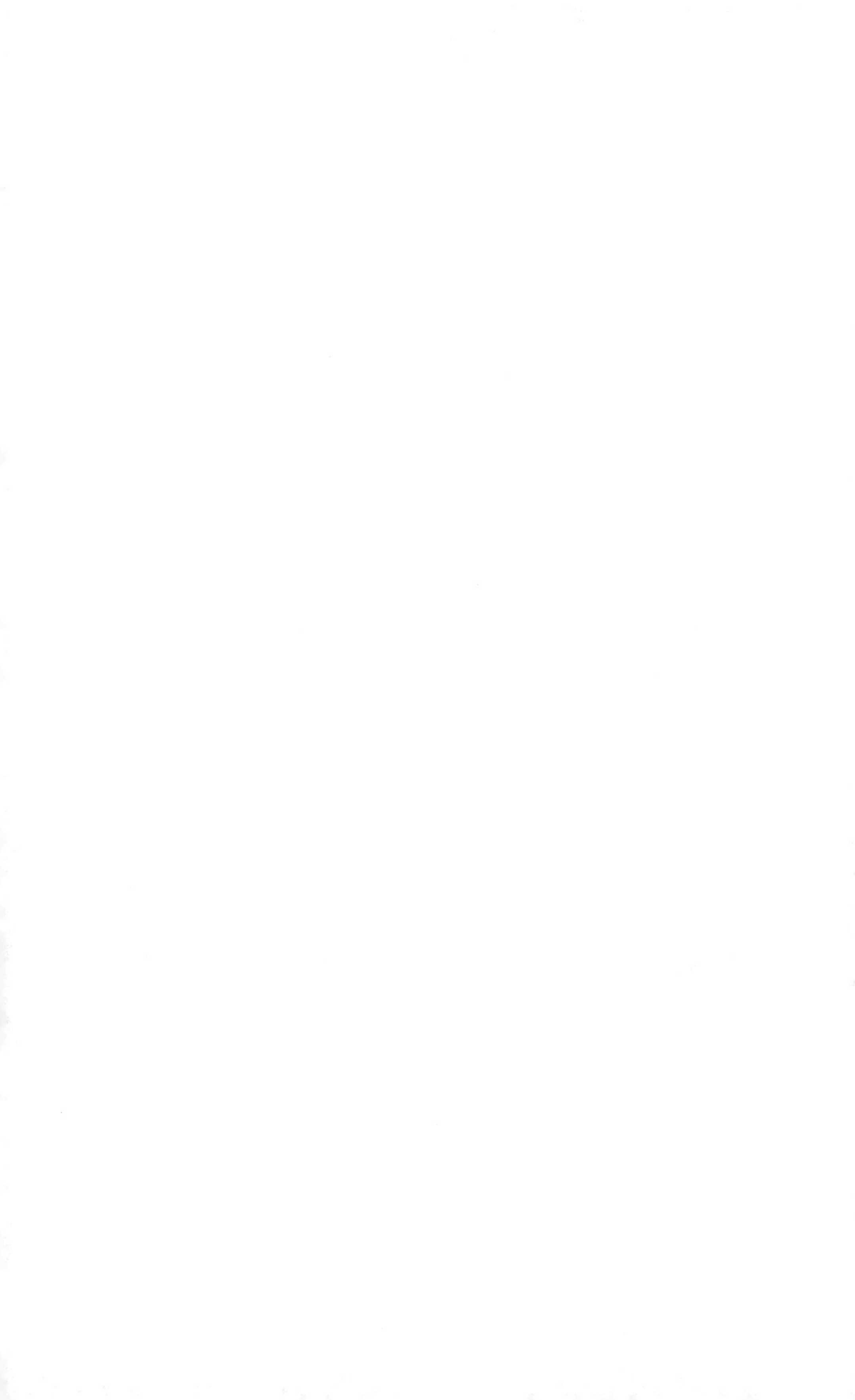

For Product Safety Concerns and Information please contact our EU representative GPSR@taylorandfrancis.com
Taylor & Francis Verlag GmbH, Kaufingerstraße 24, 80331 München, Germany

www.ingramcontent.com/pod-product-compliance
Lightning Source LLC
LaVergne TN
LVHW010857110826
845149LV00005B/1412

* 9 7 8 1 0 3 2 6 6 0 2 3 3 *